A Primer for Christian Healthcare Practice

A Primer for Christian Healthcare Practice

Prepared by
The Association of Christian Therapists

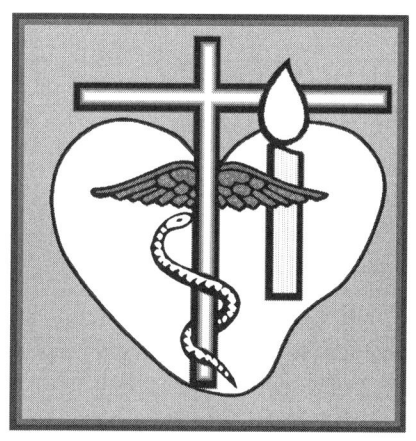

Editors:
Douglas W. Schoeninger, Ph.D.
Louis E. Lussier, M.D., Ph.D., O.S.Cam.
Kenneth M. Fung, MB, BCh, BAO, MD, FRCS
Bonita E. Lay-Oliver, B.S., MA.
Robin W. Caccese, B.S., M.T.(A.S.C.P.)

Published by
Degnon Associates, Inc.
McLean, VA

© 2001 by Association of Christian Therapists
All rights reserved

Manufactured in the United States of America

Library of Congress Control Number: 2001097466

ISBN Number: 0-9656837-3-7

For information contact:
Association of Christian Therapists
6728 Old McLean Village Drive
McLean, VA 22101
Fax: 703-556-8729
www.ACTheals.org
ACTheals@degnon.org

Published by Degnon Associated, Inc.   McLean, VA 22101

The Association of Christian Therapists

Vision Statement
To consecrate and integrate the healing professions under the Lordship of Jesus Christ.

Mission Statement
To Support, Empower and Witness to the healing professions and associates with the heart and mind of Jesus.

Purposes
Support
- To create environments in which health care professionals and associates can:
  1. grow spiritually,
  2. experience physical, mental, emotional, relational & spiritual healing,
  3. establish mutually and spiritually supportive relationships with other health care professionals and associates.

Empower
- To provide education and training in traditional and contemporary Christ-centered healing practices and in releasing the gifts of the Holy Spirit,
- To encourage and facilitate the ongoing development of leading edge Christian healing interventions.

Witness
- To train and equip members in outreach and evangelization,
- To liaise, network and collaborate with individuals and organizations with similar and complementary vision and mission,
- To initiate, encourage and support scientific research dedicated to testing and demonstrating the holistic benefits of Christ-centered healing methods and techniques,
- To creatively impact the field of integrative medicine with Christian spirituality.

The Association of Christian Therapists (ACT) began in August 1975, at Mount St. Augustine Apostolic Center in Staten Island, New York. As a group of healthcare professionals gathered to pray, study the Word of God and share Holy Eucharist, they received a vision for the consecration of their disciplines to God. This vision also called for a fellowship of men and women in the physical, mental and spiritual health care fields to make a radical commitment to the person of Jesus Christ and his mission for wholeness and holiness through prayer in the healing professions. One foundational prophetic word concerning the vision of ACT states,

> *REDEEM MY PEOPLE ... in your hospitals, in your clinics, in your offices, make them Mine. Let Me care for them, and bring them health beyond healing. Let Me care for you and bring you to health, wholeness, and holiness. Give Me your professional skills, and your credentials. Yield them to My authorization. Consecrate them to My name, for My glory and I will be glorified in My healing work.*

Mission Statements for ACT Publications

ACT seeks to develop and publish teaching about and witness to the healing power and presence of Jesus Christ through the Holy Spirit in the health and mental health professions and healing ministries. In doing this:

1. To help those committed to and practicing Christian Healing to deepen the centering and transforming of their theologies, theories, spiritual understandings and practices and professional therapies and conduct in Jesus Christ.
2. To witness to those who do not yet know of Jesus' healing power and presence, revealing God's love through the indwelling of the Holy Spirit.
3. To help reveal the mutual and reciprocal value of scientific inquiry informed by Christian faith and Christian faith informed by scientific inquiry.
4. To root wholistic care in deepening holiness.
5. To help unite healing and health with salvation and redemption.
6. To encourage the release of fresh vision and to stimulate creative contributions to healing and wholeness at all levels.
7. To reveal the resurrection of Jesus Christ our Lord and Savior at the heart of life and healing from the center of our cells and biological systems to the working of our psyches, the reaches of our spirits and in the restoration and transformation of familial, communal, corporate, international and environmental relationships.
8. To facilitate our understanding of the healing and uniting of all levels of being and relationship in Jesus Christ who is redeeming all creation.

Preface

The Association of Christian Therapists (ACT) is a unique Christian organization that embraces all disciplines of the health care professions as well as associates in healing ministries. In the midst of this diversity as health care professionals and as Christians, ACT members are united by believing in the healing presence and power of Jesus Christ, and by acknowledging the patient/client as a spiritual human being, made in the image of God.

During the past 25 years, many ACT members have been on the leading edge of developing and integrating Christian spiritual healing into their clinical professional work as medical doctors, nurses, psychiatrists, psychologists, social workers, psychotherapists, counselors, pastoral ministers, and allied health clinicians. This *Primer* is a presentation of some of this valuable work through specific case examples.

The *Primer* seeks to demonstrate the importance of recognizing the patient/client as a spiritual human being, revealing the power of healing prayer, and sharing how this is integrated into the different health care disciplines of massage, medicine, nursing, counseling and psychotherapy, organizational development and pastoral ministry.

This *Primer* is most timely with the recent surge of interest in spirituality and medicine. Most research studies done today in spirituality and health demonstrate this important relationship and the benefits to one's health, but they do not demonstrate how spiritual healing actually functions in the context of the medical, mental, psychological and pastoral presenting situations seen in clinical practice. ACT is making a significant contribution to the healing professions through the following case illustrations.

Each health discipline has its own unique understanding, language and approach to its specific health arena. It is the desire and hope that this *Primer* will generate further interest: to encourage others to share their experiences and encourage healthcare professions to cross the boundaries of their professional expertise and to develop a team approach, with a common clinical/spiritual language, in the treatment and healing of the patient/client.

The *Primer* contains six main sections: 1. Massage Therapy. 2. Medical Practice. 3. Nursing Practice, 4. Organizational Development, 5. Psychotherapy, and 6. Spiritual Direction and Prayer Ministry. The common denominator in all these sections is the spiritual component of the patient/client receiving care.

This *Primer* is a first step and a catalyst in the development and publication of an ACT Healing Manual that will foster an interdisciplinary team approach for the practice of Christian spiritual healing in medicine, psychology, counseling, pastoral ministries, organizational development and allied health interventions, and encourage research.

As indicated this *Primer* is a compilation of case illustrations of Christian healing prayer applied in a variety of professional contexts. The intent is to provide a set of "pictures" of how practitioners of various healing disciplines integrate prayers for healing and Christian spirituality with their particular healthcare discipline. We have asked the contributors to follow a particular outline in formatting their material. However we did not want this to be overly constrictive so encouraged them each to use it but also to adapt it to their needs. The result is a variety of experiences and forms of expression; those comfortable and sensible to the contributors themselves.

The goal of the *Primer* is to instruct by example. Thus each chapter will include a case illustration(s) of the integration of healing prayer and spiritual healing with a particular professional healthcare or ministry context.

The outline we used to guide contributors is as follows:
1) Title - Create a title that focuses the theme of this illustration.
2) Practitioner: Name, degrees, training, then a brief discussion of your journey of integrating healing prayer and spiritual healing with your healthcare practice.
3) Context: Description of the professional or ministry context of this illustration.
4) Goal: The therapeutic goal of this case illustration.
5) Theory/Theology: Very brief outline of the theoretical/theological frame work and assumptions that guide the author/practitioner's healing work illustrated here.
6) Methodology: Brief overview of the healing methodology.
7) Case illustration: Choose a case that well illustrates the author's integrative process.
    - Patient/client's significant history, diagnosis, symptomatology
    - Description of the clinical, diagnostic and healing interventions and processes as they were lived in this particular case. This may include one particular meeting or a course of meetings over time.
        a. Beginning - getting started.
        b. Midcourse interventions, process, responses.
        c. Concluding steps/process.
        d. Outcomes: Short-term; Long-term
8) Discussion: Added concepts/theory/theology/spirituality that further clarifies the case and method illustrated.
9) References
10) Key Words.

Our purpose with case illustrations is to demonstrate by example, including the example of each practitioner's life journey in this integrative work, as well as the example of their integrative thinking and applications. We also have tried to cover a range of healing disciplines to be both relevant to a

Preface

broad range of fields and to demonstrate the tremendous variety of styles and contexts. Jesus is present to us and to our clients and patients where we are, through what we do, where we meet others who are seeking beneficial care.

In all, we desire to reveal the heart of Jesus and his healing presence and intention. Imperfect as we each are and imperfect as our integrative thinking and applications are, the heart and mind of Jesus shines through. He uses our prayer and our desire to minister in his name to work his healing for his people through our inspired yet limited understandings and ways.

This *Primer* is the second publication in a larger context of development which we are calling the *ACT Healing Manual,* a compilation of healing resources geared to the healthcare disciplines that will make many kinds of material, bibliographies, theological and spiritual insights, methodologies etc. available for purchase. *ACT's Healing Manual* will be an ongoing developing (written, audio and video) collection of resources about Christian healing as applied in the many different healthcare disciplines. It will be made available for purchase by order, through our web site and newsletter.

Already completed is a cumulative and topical index (a 50 page booklet) of the *Journal of Christian Healing* articles (Volumes 1-22, #1&2) that is available at: www.ACTheals.org or by contacting Robin Caccese at: Phone: 610-582-5571 or email: rcaccese@talon.net. The *Journal of Christian Healing* (published by ACT through 2000) is a rich repository of *Healing Manual* material being made accessible through the *Healing Manual* process by creating this content index.

We hope you will enjoy this *Primer,* and be whetted to anticipate subsequent publications.

Table of Contents

The Association of Christian Therapists   i

Preface   iii

Massage Therapy
    1. Mary Faith Metz, L.M.T.
       God's Love Through Touch   3

Medical Practice
    2. Kenneth Fung, M.D.
       A Christian Clinical Medical Approach   9
    3. Tom Newman, M.D.
       Approaching Prayer in the Medical Setting   31
    4. Len Sperry, M.D., Ph.D.
       Integrating Medical, Psychotherapeutic and Prayer Modalities: A Case Study   39

Nursing Practice
    5. Bernice M. DeBoer, R.N., B.S.N.
       Parish Nursing in Another Faith Tradition   47
    6. Mary Jane Linn, C.S.J., R.N., Matthew Linn, S.J. and Dennis Linn, S.J.
       Healing the Dying   51
    7. Gill McLean, B.S.N.
       Compassion and the Christian Nurse   59
    8. Catherine M. Meadows, R.N.
       Healing Rites and Rituals for Nursing Care in a Changed World   65

Organizational Development
    9. Bonita Lay-Oliver, B.S., M.A.
       Healing An Organization: A Case Study   75

Psychotherapy Practice
    10. Karen Kozica Cichon, Ph.D.
       Relational Presence and the Eternal Perspective   93
    11. Georgiana G. Rodiger, Ph.D.
       The Miracle of Therapy: Finding a New Way of Being   101
    12. Joseph Scerbo, S.A., Ph.D.
       An Overview of a Spirit-Directed Therapy Session   125

13. Douglas Schoeninger, Ph.D.
Grandfather's Fear 145
14. Charles Zeiders, Psy.D. and Julie Wegryn, M.A.
Forgiveness and Healing the Repetition Compulsion 155

Spiritual Direction and Prayer Ministry
15. Louis Lussier, M.D., Ph.D., O.S.Cam.
A Generational Nightmare 167
16. Robert McGuire, S.J., M.Th.
Jesus Christ the Ultimate Healer:
Adult Child of the King (ACOK) 175
17. Robert Sears, S.J., Ph.D.
Healing as Restoration of God's Original Intent 183
18. James Wheeler, S.J.
Why Have You Forsaken Me? 199

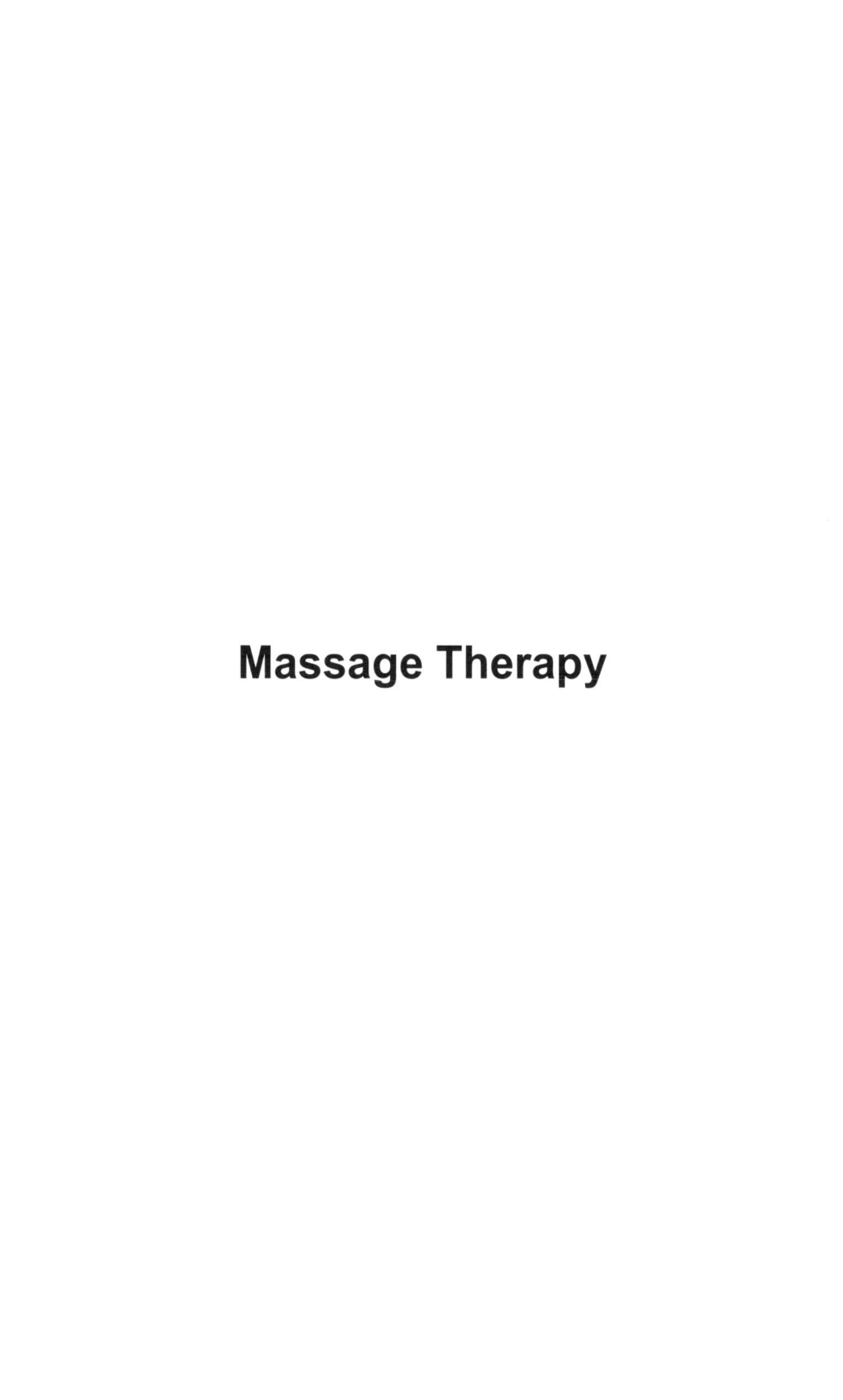

Massage Therapy

Chapter 1
God's Love Through Touch

Mary Faith Metz, L.M.T.
314-C S. Jefferson St.
Waterford, WI 53185-4252

Practitioner

Mary Faith Metz, L.M.T. completed a 500 hour course in Swedish massage at the Milwaukee School of Massage. She has been doing massage professionally part-time for 3 ½ years and in May, 2000 began doing massage therapy full-time. Mary Faith needs only to complete two more weekends of study to become certified in Neuromuscular Therapy. She is the owner of *MFM MASSAGE*. She currently treats clients at the Alumni Clinic of the Milwaukee School of Massage. She also has an office at the St. Francis Retreat Center in Burlington, WI and works two days at *The Fontana Spa* in Fontana, WI.

Journey of Integration

Following one of life's major setbacks relatively early in my adult life, someone told me of a retreat weekend. I went to that Catholic Charismatic *Life in the Spirit* weekend and things have not been the same since. That weekend began my journey into the love and healing heart of God the Father.

Several years later I was asked to be on a prayer team after our Sunday night prayer meetings at my home parish. Since then, for eighteen years, I have been praying with and for people as their needs have been brought to my attention. I am a member of the Archdiocesan Catholic Charismatic Renewal Intercessors Group in Milwaukee as well as being in the Archdiocesan Word Gift ministry.

As long as I can remember, I was always massaging some body (no pun intended), wanting to help others relax. So, I decided to go to school for massage training. Giving a massage to a person is an acceptable way to touch someone and in the process I integrate prayer, whether aloud or in silence. My touch can be a way of letting people be seen and acknowledged without being judged.

All of the massage oils I use have had Blessed Oil blended in them. Thirty minutes before my first session of the day, I bless and anoint the room and pray for myself and each client. The main prayer is that my hands become those of God/Jesus. Early on in my career my prayers with clients were always said silently. Since stepping out on my own, I have begun verbalizing prayers, openly asking Jesus to be present during the session. I have witnessed gnarled hands being straightened, joy returning to clients faces and less labored walking by some. I truly believe that our physical, mental and spiritual selves need to be in harmony with each other for wholeness. So, as I physically touch my clients I pray to also be used in bringing forth this harmony. As I am massaging I constantly pray and may envision the healing process, receive a word of knowledge (insight) or just know the words to say to someone.

Goal
In all three cases I am presenting, bringing about harmony in the entire person is the main goal. There is more to massaging a person than just rubbing muscles, improving circulation and relaxation.

Theory/Theology
Having prayed with people for so many years, I still find myself at a loss of words, awestruck that the Father would use me, a sinner, as he has when I do massage. The Bible is just full of the Lord Jesus and his apostles laying hands on people for healing. A few passages include:

Matthew 19:13-15, Jesus and the Children.
Mark 5:23-24; 8:23-25; 16:18, the Daughter of Jairus, The Blind Man at Bethsaida, The Command of the Risen Jesus to the Apostles.
Luke 4:40; 13:11;13, A Number of Cures and The Woman Who was All Bent Over.
Acts 5:12-16; 19:11-12, Cures by the Apostles, Cures by St. Paul.
Hebrews 6:2; 10:31, The Doctrine of Laying On Hands.

In doing massage, I am professionally permitted to touch another person who might otherwise not let themselves be touched, thus opening a door for the Father to touch them, to heal them and to bring their entire being into harmony.

Case Illustrations
Case #1
JoAnn's husband had committed suicide. She was the one who found him in their driveway. Earlier that week she had canceled her appointment with me, but when I called to see how she was doing, she asked me to reinstate her appointment. She said that she needed a massage. Her chief complaint was that she felt *very* tense and that every time she closed her eyes, even with a quick blink, she would *see* her husband lying there in the driveway.

Soon after starting our session, I began inwardly seeing her husband lying on the driveway. I paused and asked her if that was what she was seeing. I suspected she was because of the muscle tone and tenseness I was feeling in her face. Her reply was, "Yes." I asked if we could pray and again she said, "Yes." I kept my hands on her shoulders, gently massaging them, and then cradling her head in my hands, praying out loud. As I prayed, I imagined Jesus walking down the hill of the driveway. I then asked her to envision Jesus entering this scene and going up to her and giving her a hug. When she told me she could see Jesus there, I just prayed in tongues silently.

After about 20 minutes, I sensed that I could ask her what happened. Her muscles had begun to relax and soften. She said that she not only saw Jesus come and give her a hug, but that he also went over to her husband, stood him up and hugged him. Then she watched Jesus carry her husband to heaven. I continued praying that the healing be sealed and in no way be taken from her. As I continued giving her the massage, her tears flowed occasionally. Subsequently she no longer sees the horrible sight of her husband lying on the driveway when she closes her eyes, but rather sees Jesus there hugging him. As she tells it, many family and friends came to her and prayed with her, but no one had prayed for Jesus to meet her in the scene on the driveway.

Case #2
A psychotherapist had come to the Spa for a massage. As we talked and I found out what she did professionally. We got onto the topic of praying with clients. She was very excited about the idea, especially since she worked in a Christian office. One thing led to another in our conversation and she mentioned that she and her husband had for many years tried to become pregnant and that they were very excited when pregnancy finally happened. As I continued massaging her, I kept praying that I would be used in whatever way the Lord wanted. Then Jane revealed that she had miscarried the child and was really angry but said, "I don't want to go there." At that moment I knew that I was called to pray for her in this pain. I prayed in silence out of respect for her request. I continued to massage her and she just kept talking about her loss, which I let her do, figuring I was just to listen. Then she began sharing how the pastor that celebrated the funeral Mass had cried for them. I was touched by the compassion of this man and out of my mouth came, "You know, Jesus wept too." She asked me to repeat that, which I did and she cried. I then allowed her silence for 45 minutes, ending the massage and just being present in the room with her until it was time to end the session. When she came out of the massage room she apologized profusely for crying saying, "I have never cried like that before."

She left that day and I have not seen nor heard from her since. I do continue praying for her, that the Lord will finish the healing he began that day.

Case #3

I received a call from a new client wanting massage because she had very sore feet, shoulder and neck problems. She explained that she worked 5 days a week standing and sitting on cement flooring for eight hours at a time. In my initial session I found a severe case of hammer toes. At rest, her toes were severely bent over each other. I prayed silently as I massaged her that first time, since it was *obvious* the healing she needed. We agreed to meet once a month for the next six months. After three sessions I had not seen much improvement in her toes so I silently asked the Lord what was going on. The next time I worked with her my mind became flooded with the color red. So, I asked her if the color meant anything special to her. She said, "No." So I left it at that. This was about 4 months into our agreed 6 months of sessions. I just prayed that the Lord would reveal to her what the red color referred to. At the end of the session, as I was packing up my equipment to leave, Carla said that she knew what it was. She had had an experience with someone and was *really* mad at him. In fact, as she told me about this experience, her face became very flushed. So, I prayed with her that she be willing to forgive the person. During each of her massages, I had spent extra time working on her feet. In the last two sessions, after her sharing of this anger and our praying for the willingness to forgive, her feet showed dramatic changes. She now can walk further and longer without pain and her toes are straight.

Discussion

And so, in awe, I see how the Lord is working/acting through me and I pray: "Father, Daddy, help me to always keep my eyes focused on your face and your will. Keep my ears open to your voice and my spirit quickened by your prompting to do or say something. It is not I that does any of this - it is *you*. May I remain forever mindful that it is *you*. Continue to change my human hands into your hands bringing your Love, Healing, Peace and Presence to others lives. Amen.

Medical Practice

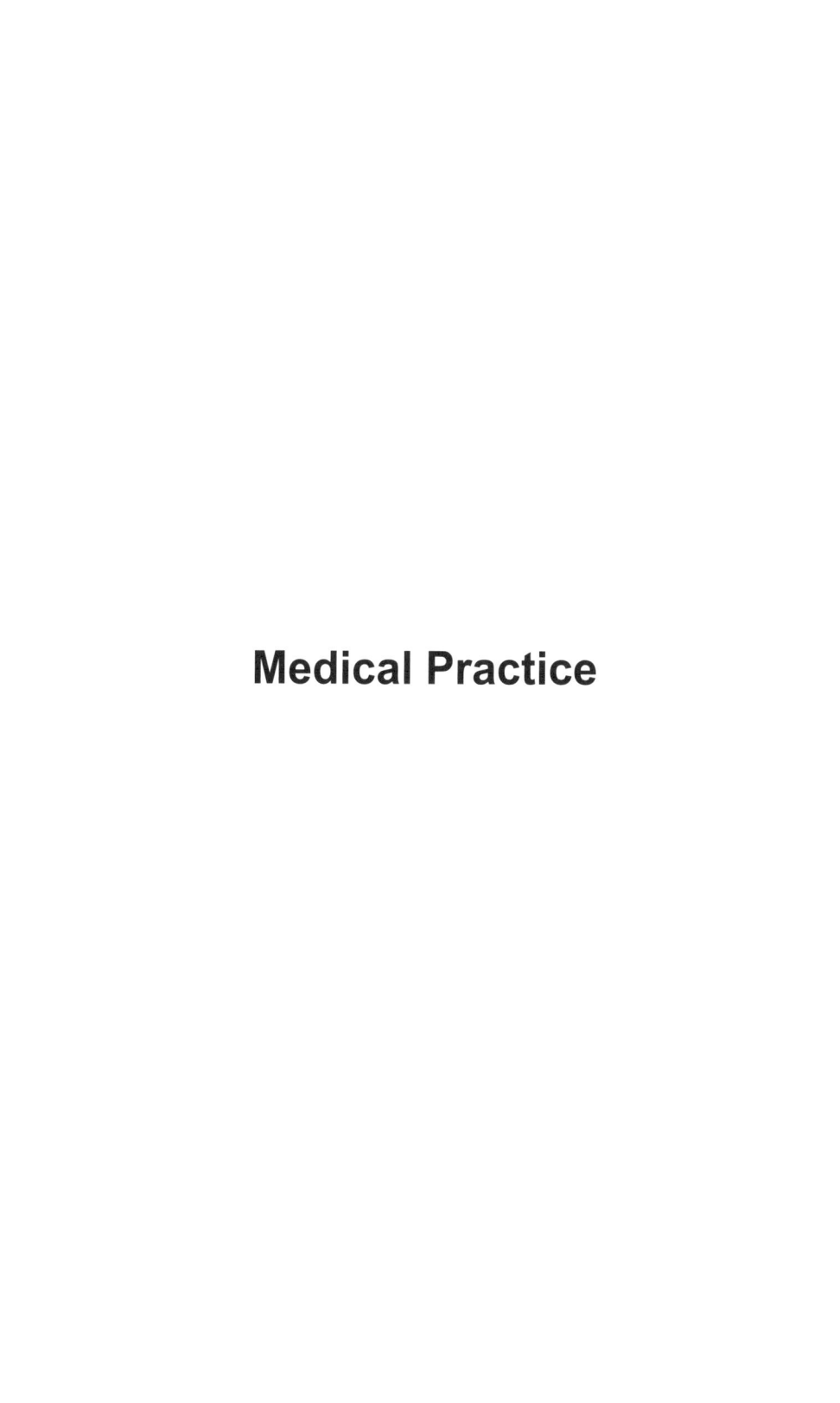

Chapter 2

A Christian Clinical Medical Approach

Kenneth M. Fung, M.B., B.Ch., B.A.O., M.D., F.R.C.S.
26 Farmington Crescent
Agincourt, Ontario, M1S 1G1, Canada

Practitioner

Dr Kenneth Fung is a practicing Christian family physician, counsellor, and psychotherapist, who integrates the spirituality of Christian healing into his professional work. Dr. Fung was born in Trinidad and studied Medicine at the National University of Ireland in Gallway. He graduated in 1961 and obtained his FRCS* in England. He became an Associate Professor of Surgery in the University of the West Indies and practiced general and thoracic surgery in England and Trinidad, before immigrating to Canada in 1970. He worked on a research fellowship in thoracic surgery at the University of Toronto before establishing a Family Practice. In 1980 he joined the Association of Christian Therapists (ACT) and embarked on a journey that modified his personal and professional life. His practice is registered as The Christian Medical Centre, offering his patients total medical care through the integration of traditional medicine and all forms of Christian healing. The latter includes healing prayer, Christian psychotherapy and counselling. He served as President of the Association of Christian Therapists from 1993-1995.

Journey of Integration

When I was a young resident doctor in Ireland it was not traditional for a doctor to pray with his patients. At that time, if I thought a patient was dying, I felt that it was my responsibility as a Christian physician to make sure that the priest saw the person before he died. Later, in Trinidad, I was working in a hospital that did not have the best facilities. The hospital administrator's 17 year old son developed a cardiac arrest. I was in his house trying to resuscitate him and for all practical purposes I thought he was dead. It took us over an hour to get his heart beating and we did not have any defibrillators. All we had was manpower. We were trying to do external cardiac massage, to get a carotid pulse and to get an open airway. While we were doing this people were looking in through the windows. Many heard about this and came. In the midst of all of this a priest came and began blessing us with Holy Water. He kept saying , "Say, 'Jesus, Mary and Joseph, I love you'." I was thinking, "What is this guy doing here?" After about an hour, to my surprise, the patient's heart began to beat. I was then worried that he would have had brain damage from this cardiac arrest. Then he started shouting,

---

* Fellow of the Royal College of Surgeons

"Jesus, Mary and Joseph, I want to live." I looked at that as good, but I didn't see anything much more than that. I thought I did my part and the priest did his part. Sometime later I prayed for a patient with cancer. She had not been doing very well. I thought she was going to die that night so I called the priest. The priest gave her the anointing that used to be called Extreme Unction. The priest later said that she was in peace and on her way to heaven. I thanked him. The next morning I came and found her sitting up in bed. She was discharged within a few days. At that time it never occurred to me that this was a miracle of God's healing love. In medicine we would say that maybe it was a remission and these things happen.

When I first came to Canada I was doing thoracic surgery at the University of Toronto. In order to make a little extra money for my family, I opened up an office to do Family Practice. To my surprise, I discovered a relationship with patients I never had as a specialist. It made me realize that they put a trust in me. That trust bothered me a bit. I realized that if they were going to trust me like that, I had to respond to them in some way. This made me look into my own personal life. I discovered that there were fears in me - fears of what people might say, of what might happen.

I also began to see that a lot of the problems of patients who came in were not purely medical problems. There were a lot of other underlying issues. This was also the time that I began to become involved in the charismatic renewal in my church. I was experiencing God's love in a new way and beginning to see things differently. I realized that it would help my patients if they could understand God's healing love. I discovered that it was okay to pray with a patient, but I was afraid to do it. Initially, the most I could do was point to the ceiling and say to a patient, "Do you know the guy up there?" The patient would look up to the ceiling. I know that they knew what I was talking about. I wanted to pray with them, but I didn't have the courage.

A woman from the Salvation Army came to me because she had been depressed for years and had not been helped by other doctors. She claimed that she was *Born Again*. However, she would only go to church if she felt happy that day, so she could smile and everyone could see that she was filled with the Spirit. If she was depressed, she would not go to church. She was afraid that people might think that something was wrong with her. I wanted to pray with her, but I didn't have the courage. One day I said to her, "God will never heal you if you don't learn how to go to him as your true self." She walked out of the office very sad. I felt bad because I knew that part of the reason I said that was because I was projecting onto her my fear of wanting to pray and not being able to do so. That week she found herself in the kitchen saying, "Lord, I'm giving you your last chance. You better do something or else." Then she felt a deep peace come over her and she felt renewed. This excited her and she came to tell me the story. Since she was so excited, I asked her what she wanted to do. She said, "I just want to praise God." Without thinking, I said, "Why don't we do that?" She grabbed my hand and held it up in the air and was praising God. I was thinking, "If my secretary comes in the office, what will happen!" God was merciful and kept the door closed, but the experience broke the ice for me to find the courage to begin praying with patients.

At the same time my patients began to bring me things like a little desk-mounted crucifix or leave little cards with Bible quotations in my office. Then patients would begin to say, "Doc, I didn't know you were *Born Again* or a *Christian*." The little cards were their signs telling me that they were Christian also. These things were giving me little boosts. I realized that really, Jesus was coming to me through my patients. They were the ones who were really teaching me. This kind of learning became so important to me that I was afraid to go to any of the official university courses because I thought they would really confuse my growing faith. God was teaching me through my patients.

At a lecture I heard a priest psychiatrist say, "If you don't know how to renew your faith, a good way is to read scripture." He said that a good scripture passage was Isaiah 43. I had never heard of Isaiah 43. The priest said that wherever the word *you* or *Israel* appeared, to substitute one's own name for it.

I often find that after I learn some new healing truth, a patient will come in and the thought of what I just learned will come up in my mind. A woman came in who was having neck pains. She had been to nine doctors who had all prescribed pills. I was thinking that I had better not give her pills. At the same time I asked her how she was coping at night. She said that she did not sleep and she guessed, "That God wanted her to stay up all night and pray." I replied, "I don't know about your God, but I can't imagine my God giving me pains in my neck to get me to stay up all night and pray. I'd be miserable the next day." I thought of Isaiah 43. I told her I had just heard a priest psychiatrist say that one way of healing was to renew your faith, by reading scripture. I asked her if she would like to try this. She gave me a strange look, but said "Ok." I wrote Isaiah 43 on my prescription pad and gave it to her. I wondered if she thought I was crazy. A week later she came back and I asked her how she was feeling. She said, "Awful. I haven't stopped crying since I read that passage. Even when my husband died, I never cried like this." I asked the Lord to tell me what to say. I was thinking that she spoke of tears, water, so I said, "Maybe God is washing you clean." Then she began telling me her whole history. Apparently she was an alcoholic. She concluded, "Was I not stupid?" I asked her why she thought that. She said, "He was always there, but I kept looking the opposite way." I asked her who was always there. She said, "Jesus." I asked her how she felt. She said, "I feel so empty." I asked her what she wanted to do. She said, "I guess I'm going to fill it with his love." The way that she said it, I wanted to say like Jesus did, "Woman, your faith has healed you. Go in peace to love and serve the Lord." The pain left her. That was over 15 years ago.

Little experiences like these were happening to me. They gave me confidence to continue integrating my Christian faith and prayer into my medical practice.

Context

The context is a family practice medical office called The Christian Medical Centre in which I utilize a novel clinical approach that integrates Christian spirituality with clinical medical and counseling practice. I call this approach *The Christian Clinical Medical Model.*

Goal

The main goal in my practice of Christian medicine is to treat every patient as a spiritual human being and to demonstrate to those patients, whose symptoms persist in spite of medical treatment, that their symptoms or illness can have an underlying spiritual basis. This is especially so when all tests and investigations are normal. Finally I offer healing prayer as part of my treatment.

Theory/Theology

The present clinical medical, psycho/social model of medicine does not acknowledge spirituality as a causative factor in the etiology and symptomatology of illness, sickness and disease. It only sees the patient as a human, physical and psychological being, and not as a spiritual human being. Conversely, the patient may not be aware of the role their spirituality may play in the underlying root cause of their symptoms and illness. This even applies to persons who have Christian faith and believe in the power of healing prayer.

It is my opinion that if the patient's spirituality is adversely affected, i.e. *broken*, spiritual stress may develop and could become a major underlying and undetected causal factor in the patient's physical, emotional and mental symptoms. This is especially so when all the medical tests and investigations are normal. Healing of a *broken* spirit, often in combination with medical treatment and psychotherapy, is integral in helping to restore the patient to full health, of body, mind and spirit.

This Christian clinical medical approach enables the physician to integrate spiritual healing with medical science and psychology. It does not impose religious beliefs on the patient, but respects the patient's religious views.

{This process is what I think of as the true *art* of Christian medicine.}

The Nature of the Human Person and Human Brokenness:
A Spiritual Medical Psycho-Social Theory of Illness

Following is an outline of how I view the nature of the human person and human brokenness, spiritually, psychologically and physically.

Spiritual:
1. We are human beings made in the image and likeness of God.
   "*God created man in his Image; in the divine Image he created him, male and female he created them*" (Genesis 1:27).
   "*You created every part of me; you put me together in my mother's womb*" (Ps. 139:13).
2. We are spiritual human beings.
   "*God's Spirit joins himself to our spirit*" (Romans 8:16).
3. We are children of God, free to become what we were created to be.
   "*His love is so great that we are called God's children*" (1 John 3:1).
4. As spiritual human beings, we desire to do good, to love, etc.
   "*The spirit produces love, joy, peace, patience, goodness, faithfulness, kindness, humility and self-control*" (Galatians 5:22-23).

Psychological:
1. As a spiritual human being, made in the image and likeness of God, we are affirmed in our true identity as a child of God, with our unique gifts and talents.
2. As a spiritual human being the child needs to be in relationship and affirmed in the spirit of God's love in order to grow, mature, and develop into the authentic person the child was created to be.
3. Lack of affirming love and loving meaningful relationships could adversely affect this spiritual identity development. This could start in the womb.
4. Adverse enviromental and social factors could also affect the child's spiritual, emotional and mental development.
5. The younger the child experiences these adversities, the more likely the negative feelings of not being lovable or worthy will develop, with adverse psychological behavioural traits.
6. If these negative feelings prevail, it could distort the child's sense of his identity, as being unlovable, not good enough, worthless, etc., or the contrary, to be superior, invincible, better than, etc.
7. The child may eventually come to believe these negative feelings as true [*False Belief*], and therefore see his identity as a person to be

defective, or to be invincible [*the Lie*].
8. This causes the spirit to be traumatised [*Broken Spirit*].
9. Rather than live in the light of the truth, he lives in the darkness of *the Lie*.
10. *The Lie* in turn creates *false needs* to prove one's self as lovable, worthwhile, invincible, etc.
11. These false needs create *unrealistic expectations* of self, other, and God, that are never met, resulting in repeated disappointments.
12. The cycle of repeated dissappointments results in mixed emotions of anger, guilt, and fear, reinforcing *the Lie* and the shame of unworthiness.
13. This condition creates stress. This stress is called *Spiritual Stress*.

Medical:
1. Spiritual Stress, follows the same neuro-chemical and neuro-endocrine pathways of any other form of stress.
2. Spiritual stress in turn triggers the physiologic stress hormone [CRH-ACTH-Cortisol] release and behavioral response via the hypothalamo-pituitary-adrenal axis, and the sympathetic nervous system produces epinephrine and nor-epinephrine [CRH—corticotropin release hormone and ACTH—adeno corticotropic hormone].
3. If the spiritual stress is corrected, then the stress hormone response is shut off and returns to its normal base line levels (McEwen, 1998).
4. If the spiritual stress is prolonged and becomes chronic, four situations could arise (Fulgosi, July, 2000):
   a. Bouts of repeated and recurrent stressors;
   b. Inability to shut off the stress responses due to the reduced negative feed back effects of cortisol (This could lead to memory loss from failure to turn off the release of the excitatory amino acids [glutamate]);
   c. Diminished or inadequate response of the hypothalamo-pituitary-adrenal axis to generate enough cortisol. (This can result in compensatory increase in the secretion of the inflammatory cytokines, a possible cause of the symptoms of chronic fatigue syndrome and fibromyalgia.);
   d. Inability to cope or adapt to recurrent stress.
5. Chronic prolonged spiritual stress combined with socio-economic stress and genetic disease factors could have a serious effect on the immune and endocrine systems, as well as on cardio-vascular heart disease, degenerative brain disorders, metabolic and immune disorders (House, 1990).

Conclusion:
1. The most likely *underlying cause* of physical, emotional, amd mental symptoms, when all medical tests are normal, is *Spiritual Stress*. ✗
2. The deepest underlying *root cause* of a patient's *Spiritual Stress* is their *Broken Spirit*.
3. Persistence of spiritual stress together with genetic, familial, psychological, and enviromental factors, could eventually lead to illness, sickness, and disease.
4. Healing of the broken spirit, often in combination with medical treatment and psychotherapy, helps to restore the patient to full health of body, mind and spirit.
5. The *Spiritual Stress* is replaced with inner peace, love, and freedom, as the patient comes into the fullness of the truth in his identity as a spiritual human being.
6. Freedom to become one's true authentic self with one's unique gifts and talents is restored with harmony of body, mind and spirit.
7. I call this process the *Art* of Christian Medicine and Christian Psychotherapy.

Methodology
The Challenge
1. How can I demonstrate to my patient that their symptoms or illness can have an underlying spiritual basis? This is especially so when all tests and investigations are normal, in spite of persistent symptoms and the patient's condition not improving with medical treatment.
2. How can I offer prayer to my patient for healing? Christian healing prayer can lead to spontaneous healing, especially physical and mental healing. In my experience, healing prayer, in conjunction with medication, psychotherapy, and patient compliance (a patient committed to making necessary changes), are often required in combination for healing of illness.

The Objectives
1. To help the patient *become aware,* in a clinical professional manner, that their symptoms/illness may have a spiritual basis, without imposing the physician's religious beliefs on the patient.
2. To help *identify* the *Lie* and the *Secret* (false self) in the patient's self-identity.
3. To help the patient *recognize*, the *Broken Spirit* and the *Spiritual Stress* within.
4. To *demonstrate* to the patient the relationship between spiritual stress and illness.

5. To *treat* the patient with medical scientific knowledge and skills.
6. To *offer* the patient healing prayer and to discover the truth about self and God.
7. To *affirm* and *empower* the patient's authentic self, unique gifts and talents.

Assessing Breakdowns and Promoting Healing:
The Christian Clinical Medical Model
The Christian Clinical Medical Model sees the patient as a spiritual human being and is divided into four aspects for clinical purposes:
1. Spiritual [identity, faith belief],
2. Psychological [affective, cognitive, connative],
3. Medical [physical, emotional, mental],
4. Social/lifestyle.

These four aspects are assessed in four modules:

Spiritual Module: This module could be likened to taking a spiritual history. It involves helping the patient to discover his/her perceived identity of self that he/she believes to be true, based on his/her early childhood life experiences (spiritual legacy). I acknowledge this belief as the patient's Spiritual *faith belief* of self. I also do the same process to uncover the patient's spiritual faith belief in an image of God or the higher power.

I next encourage the patient to review his/her identity as a *spiritual human being*, made in the image and likeness of God. This process allows the patient to rediscover the truth about self, the gift of being an authentic person with unique gifts of God's love and special natural talents. It also enables the patient to discover if there are any discrepancies in his/her identity, between what the patient believes to be true, and what he/she feels is true for any person made in the image and likeness of God. Is the patient's faith belief of self true or false? Similarly, is the patient's image of God true or false?

In almost every case there are false beliefs of self and of God - the *Lie*. These develop out of the patient's spiritual legacy and the patient's own wrong doing, i.e. where they have failed to love God and to love their neighbor as themselves. False beliefs of self and God result in a *broken spirit*.

Healing prayer is required for the healing of the *broken spirit* and enables the patient to reclaim his or her authentic identity with their unique gifts and talents.

Psychological Module: This module could be likened to taking a psychological history. It relates to the free will, the emotions and feelings, the cognitive and connative functions, and the behavioral characteristics of the patient. It also involves the personality formation of the patient, in relation to self-perceptions, attitudes, coping behaviors, motives, and expectations of self and other. These psychological factors enable the patient to make choices and decisions. They could be right or wrong, and are determined or strongly influenced by the patient's spiritual belief of self and God, i.e. operating out of the *lie* or the *truth*.

If the decisions or the behaviors of the patient are influenced by the *lie*, i. e. the false identity, then the patient operates out of an identity that is defective, the *false belief*, which creates *false needs* to prove the self, with *unrealistic expectations* of self, other, and God. Behavioral coping which strives for a false need I call the *Secret*. This results in recurrent disappointments, with a revolving cycle of mixed emotions of anger, guilt, and fear. Self-esteem, self-worth, self-confidence, and self-respect progressively diminish. I call this recurrent cycle *negative spiritual stress*, which activates the stress hormonal response via the hypothalamic-pituitary-adrenal axis in an excessive manner.

If the decision or the behavior of the patient is influenced by the *truth*, i.e. the authentic identity, then the patient operates out of a true identity, with natural gifts and talents. This allows the patient to be free and to become the true authentic person. There are no disappointments, as the patient learns to accept life as it comes, can acknowledge a mistake if there is one, learn from it, and make the best of life, trusting in God. This results in *positive spiritual stress* that affirms and empowers the patient to live life to the fullest!

In this area of therapy, I identify those parts of the patient that are most weak, hurting and vulnerable. This is followed with healing prayer for the memories of the hurts and the woundedness. Christian psychotherapy involves seeking God's wisdom. The patient is invited to renew his or her faith belief, as well as to forgive self, and the other, and to receive God's healing love. This is an ongoing process and not a one-time treatment.

Medical Health Module: I see this aspect as having two facets:
  1) Health
This section relates to the effects of continued *negative spiritual stress* on the emotional, mental and physical aspects of the patient, that may result in physical, emotional, and mental symptoms. This process develops through the neuro-endocrine system, involving the excessive or diminished release of stress hormones via the hypothalamic, pituitary, and adrenal axis, as well as the sympathetic nervous system acting upon the target organs of the body. Some examples of stress on organic bodily functions include:
    a) *The Endocrine Organs*: thyroid hypo-function affecting body metabolism; pancreatic functioning, affecting sugar metabolism, as in diabetes; impaired function of the immune system causing low-

ered resistance to infection; and sexual/hormonal dysfunction, leading to impotency, lowered libido, dysmenorrhoea (severe menstrual pain), amenorrhoea (cessation of menstruation), etc.

b) *The Organs of the Body*: the cardio vascular system - palpitations, hypertension; the gastro-intestinal system - spastic colon, irritable bowel, nausea, indigestion, diarrhea; skin integrity - skin rashes, eczema, itchiness; muscular integrity - aches and pains, tension headaches, fibromyalgia, chronic fatigue; brain function - moderate depression, anxiety, stress disorder.

2) Medical

This section relates to disease processes involving the emotional, mental and physical aspects of the patient. e.g. heart disease, myocardial infarction, atrial fibrillation; cancer of the various organs; bone and joint diseases - rheumatoid arthritis; lung disease - asthma; metabolic diseases - Type II diabetes, hypo thyroidism; mental illnesses - clinical depression, anxiety disorders, panic attacks, bipolar depression and borderline personality disorders.

The use of medical science interventions, including medication, technology, operations, etc. is often required and necessary. I believe that disease conditions may result from the effects of the chronic spiritual stress upon the body, together with the adverse environmental and social conditions in patients who are genetically pre-disposed to certain illnesses.

Through this process the patient becomes more aware and able to understand the possible connection between the symptoms of illness and the *negative spiritual stress* of the *broken spirit*. The patient also becomes more open to healing prayer with medical treatment.

Healing prayer for underlying *spiritual stress* and a *broken spirit* may result in spontaneous healing. Often a patient's condition significantly improves after healing prayer and the patient is able to cope much better.

Social/lifestyle Module: This module could be likened to taking a social/lifestyle history. It relates to the patient's personality, behavior, coping life skills, and the ability to accept and take responsibility for the consequences in their relationships, family life, socialization, career, and finances. Again, how the patient functions will be greatly influenced by his/her spiritual beliefs of self and God, as well as the state of the patient's psychological/spiritual stress and medical health.

These four aspects of assessment help the patient to become aware of areas of weakness and dysfunction. They also enable the patient to become aware of and to understand the connection between the underlying spiritual root problem of the *broken spirit*, the *lie*, and the dysfunctional coping behavior.

Case Illustrations
Case 1. Severe Recurrent Anterior Chest Pains. Major Clinical Depression
M.A. male, age 42, eldest of three brothers, married with two children, suddenly developed acute severe anterior chest pains. At the hospital emergency unit all investigations, including his cardiogram and blood tests were normal. He was reassured and sent home. One week later his symptoms recurred and again he showed up at the emergency unit. All tests again proved negative, and he was sent home. He was now becoming very agitated as the pain persisted. "What is the cause of my pain?", he asked. He felt very vulnerable and powerless. Prior to this episode, his 14 year old son began attending high school and was unable to have lunch with him as he was accustomed to in junior high school. His wife also started a new job that involved traveling on the highway for 30 minutes. The combination of his undiagnosed chest pains, missing his son at lunch time, and fearing the worst for his wife driving on the highway, resulted in the onset of acute anxiety and clinical depression, all within a five week period. His past medical history was uneventful.

Applying the four module *Christian Clinical Medical Model* to obtain his spiritual, psychological, medical and social/lifestyle histories, I discovered:

1. *Spiritual history* - I was able to identify in his *broken spirit*, the *lie* [the false belief] he had about himself, i.e. *not good enough* in the eyes of his father, since age 10. Although Roman Catholic, he did not practice his religious beliefs and felt guilt and fear of an angry punishing God. He had remained in this guilt for 30 years. At 12 years of age, he had attempted to steal money from his grandmother, who trusted him.
2. *Psychological history* - I was able to uncover his *secret*, ie. his false need to prove he was a somebody, to overcome the *lie*. This dysfunctional behavior was accomplished by projecting himself as a very macho, cool, strong, masculine male and by pleasing others [could not say no] and approval seeking.
3. *Medical history* - Physical symptoms consisted of chest pains, insomnia, shortness of breath, tiredness. Emotional symptoms included agitation, anxiety, nervousness. Mental symptoms were anxiety and major depression.
4. *Social/lifestyle history* - The patient's relationships were based on fear and seeking approval. Family life was characterized by pleasing others, loyalty, over-protection and over-attachment. Social life went from extraversion to withdrawal. Career evolved from fulfilling hard work to painful effort at work. Financial well being initially permitted him to be generous, but now he had lost interest in giving.

Cause of chest pain: Medically, in light of all tests being normal, I believe his chest pains developed from the increased tension of his anterior chest wall and intercostal muscles. This tension was probably related to the deep emotional fears of rejection, abandonment, and death, he was experiencing. The fears exposed his own vulnerability and powerlessness. Not practicing his faith, meant he had nothing to trust in but himself, but his vulnerability and powerlessness made that difficult, and so he was unable to cope.

However, seeking the deeper root cause of his vulnerability and fears led us to the underlying *spiritual stress* that existed from his *broken spirit* and the *lie* about himself as *not good enough* and about his God, as *angry, punishing*, together with his *secret* "to prove himself," and his guilt of 30 years.

Healing: In praying together for healing of his *broken spirit*, he was able to acknowledge, accept, and forgive his father as well as himself. We also discovered his gift of compassion, and his talent as being very athletic. He made a decision to return to church, taking his family with him, and to let go of the *lie*, his *secret*, and his fears by trusting in God. In one week, he was feeling more peaceful and his chest pains had decreased. He required a low dose of anti-depressant medication for one year and now has no more pain. He may get occasional bouts of anxiety, as he continues to be transformed from the darkness of the *lie* of not being good enough into the light of the *truth* as the compassionate, caring, athletic husband and father. He has been set free to become his true authentic self. He has reconciled with his father and attends church regularly with his family. He actively plays tennis, never misses work and always has a smile on his face. He is also able to express himself more readily. These changes have been sustained for over three years.

Case 2. Severe Dysmenorrhoea and Pre Menstrual Cramps

Mrs V.A., age 42, suffered from severe dysmenorrhoea and premenstrual cramps that occurred exactly seven days before the start of each menstrual cycle for 3 years. When first seen she had already been to nine gynecologists without any success. In her medical history, I discovered that her symptoms had started following an abortion at age 39. She was very defensive and argued to justify her action to abort, by stating her age and the financial need to keep her job at that time. She was married and had two children, age 14 and 12. All gynecological and pelvic investigations were normal.

Introducing her to the Christian Clinical Medical Model, with the patient as a spiritual human being, she was able to discover her *broken spirit* and the *lie* in her life, i.e. the false belief that she was *not good enough*. She also became aware of the *spiritual stress* from her dysfunctional way of coping as a perfectionist and seeking approval, her *secret*, as only she knew the deeper motives for her actions, a deep need to be accepted. She was very critical of others.

Cause of her pain and cramps: What were the possible causes of her premenstrual and menstrual pains? Could it be they were from the chronic *spiritual stress* from her denial of guilt in having the abortion, which she eventually admitted was wrong. They may also have arisen from the deep fear linked to the severe post abortion bleeding complications, when she thought *she almost died*. These may have resulted in the reenforcement of the *lie*, i.e. the false belief that she was *not good enough*, and not being able to accept the fact that she became pregnant in spite of her perfectionist attitude in which she wanted always to be in control.

Healing: The patient admitted having a Christian faith belief, but was not practicing her faith. Also on admitting her guilt, she said she had felt, as she exerienced the complications to the abortion, "that God had a purpose and plan for her," but was never sure what that meant. We were able to choose a name for the aborted baby and praying with her through Jesus Christ, she was able to express her feelings of love and remorse to the baby, calling her by name. She had felt the baby was a girl. She was able to forgive herself, repented, and accepted Jesus, as her Lord and Savior. We also prayed for financial help to repair her home furnace, which had broken down. She made a free decision to go back to church, with her family.

Three things happened as a result of our prayers together:
1. Driving home that evening there was a severe rain storm. *She discovered her fear of driving in rain storms had vanished*. She felt a deep peace at home that night.
2. Her menstrual cycle started unexpectedly the following day, i.e. one week early *without pain!*
3. She received *a surprise* increase in salary, three months retro-active, equal to the cost of repairing the furnace, $1200!

She stated "In my 42 years, this was the best week of my entire life, Praise God!" *All of this occurred in the week following a two-hour session and she required nothing more.* She has had no premenstrual or menstrual pains since for over seven years and has never needed any medication.

Case. 3. *Severe Major Depression and Anxiety*

Mrs A. age 36, married a second time with two children, ages 3 and 5 years, developed severe major clinical depression. On her first visit, she stated she had been depressed for over nine months, and had consulted her family doctor as well as a psychiatrist. She had tried several anti-depressants but had reacted badly to these; she was now afraid to take pills. She also had not worked since that time. She was now becoming increasingly concerned as it was affecting her relationships with her husband and children, worrying how her children might be affected since her patience and tolerance were very low. She felt very guilty and feared losing her job and marriage. She was also afraid of *going out of her mind*. She had started attending a prayer group and healing Masses; these gave her some support and hope.

Introducing her to the Christian Clinical Medical Model, I was able to help her discover her *broken spirit*, and the *lie* in her life. She believed she was the *black sheep* in her family and was cursed since age 12, when she was taken by her mother to a spiritual healer, who sexually abused her. Her mother never believed her.

Although seeming happily married with two beautiful children and holding a secure job, the *lie* caused her to cope by being a perfectionist. This dysfunctional way of coping was her *secret*.

The resultant *spiritual stress* in trying to keep up to her perfectionistic expectations of her false self, was too much. She also had unrealistic expectations of her children and of her mother, reflecting her need to be accepted, and this added to the stress. These recurrent disappointments led to feelings of anger, guilt, anxiety, associated with increased feelings of poor self-worth and self-esteem. Her first marriage was a failure and she carried feelings of guilt and shame for its failure, feeling she was the eldest and role model in her family. She felt God was punishing her. All these factors led to her depression.

Healing: Over a period of nine months, with Christian cognitive and support therapy, she was able to come to know the truth about herself as the compassionate, loving, creative, athletic girl (she had been), made in the image and likeness of God, and about God as a loving, faithful, understanding Father, whom she could trust. To forgive her mother and herself was not easy, nor was agreeing to take anti-depressant medication again.

Mrs A's depression subsided with medication. She now lives in the light of the truth about herself and God. She has become free of the *lie* and is learning to love, accept, and become more of her true self each day. She has returned to work, and most of all, is now learning how to love, accept and enjoy her husband and children as they are, unconditionally, and not how she would like them to be. Her perfectionist ways are diminishing and she is coping more efficiently. At present, she remains on a very low dose of anti-depressants. She attends a weekly prayer meeting. She is now 15 months into her recovery.

Case 4. Severe Chronic Epigastric Pain and Depression

Mr. E.L. 34 ys. was brought to my office by his friend, whom he recently met at church while seeking God for help. He was suffering from intractable severe epigastric abdominal pains for seven months. He was suicidal as he could not live with the pain, could not eat a normal meal nor swallow any pills. He had been fully investigated by several gastro enterologists, with numerous X-rays, CT Scans, MRI tests plus gastroscopic and colonic examinations to no avail. The only findings were mild gastro esophageal reflux and scarring from a healed duodenal ulcer. All medications for reflux and hyperacidity had failed. He was afraid to take any pill medication as it actually made his pain worse. Anti-Depressants in the past had also failed. He had come to believe that his "stomach was so badly damaged that only an operation would help him." The specialists told him that his tests were normal and they could not find a physical cause to explain his pain.

On taking his medical history, I discovered he had attempted suicide with an overdose of 100 aspirins, eleven months before. About three months later, his epigastric pain got much more worse when he had a "few beers to celebrate his birthday." He felt guilty for drinking the beer. Prior to his suicide attempt, he was recovering from depression following two years of alcohol and drug abuse. He had been hospitalized for depression and under psychiatric therapy since then.

Family and social history revealed he was the eldest of 13 children and had suffered physical abuse from his father; his mother had a problem with her *nerves*. He left home and school at 14 years of age. At age 18, he got married, and one year later the marriage was over. He then met a girl, had a relationship that lasted a few weeks and it resulted in her becoming pregnant. He did not know he had become a father until years later. His daughter is now 16 years old, but he is unable to see her. He had not been able to work and was on welfare. He was without funds and felt very guilty and angry, " I am young, I should be able to work," he said.

On introducing him to the Christian medical model, we discovered his *broken spirit* and the *lie* in his early life, *never good enough*. He tried to satisfy his false self by *doing his thing*. This was his *secret* way. The resultant *spiritual stress* of doing his thing led to the following consequences: a broken marriage, an eighth grade education, getting a girl pregnant, alcohol and drugs, a suicide attempt, untrained without regular job. He felt he was a failure and carried tremendous guilt and anger. There was also shame, despair and a sense of hopelessness. God was not answering his prayer, in spite of his going back to church, and praying.

We also discovered that at age eight, he had sustained a very serious internal abdominal injury: while tobogganing down a slope, he collided with a chair leg partly buried in the snow. He was hospitalized for one week. His present abdominal epigastric pain was very similar.

Cause of Pain: Could there have been an subconscious relationship between his initial abdominal injury pain at eight years that justified him being in a hospital, and the present epigastric abdominal pains, that prevented him from working and taking responsibility for his health and well being? Also could the *spiritual stress* from his *secret*, i.e. *doing his thing* and his living in the darkness of the *lie* "never good enough" be factors in his pain? I also discovered he was not able to forgive himself, from all the shame of his past.

Healing: We prayed for the grace to forgive himself and others, to discover the truth about himself as the compassionate, caring, musically creative boy (he had been), and about God as a loving, faithful and merciful Father. Through cognitive and support therapy, he was able to grasp other possible causes for his pain, namely, psychosomatic. He struggled with trying to say it was all in his head. Ultimately he was able to see and understand the possible relationship between his *broken spirit*, his *lie*, his *secret*, with its consequences, and the underlying *spiritual stress* of his false self; this resulted in his severe epigastric pains, similar to his childhood pains.

He finally agreed to take medication to control his *abdominal spasms* and his anxiety. We prayed for protection from side effects of the medication. Although he took the medication with a great deal of trepidation and fear, the pain suddenly subsided after taking the pills, and he said, "I felt almost 75% cured, Thanks be to God!" He believes God has answered his prayer and has healed him, although he continues to remind me that he is not completely pain free, and has some residual fear of a relapse. Though this is a realistic concern, our faith is always in a struggle with our lived experiences.

He has continually improved since, is now eating normally, has become cheerful, hopeful, and his depression has lifted. His self-esteem has increased, he has started playing his guitar again, and attends daily Mass. He has not complained of pain since and continues to take his medication.

This whole process took four one-hour sessions, over two weeks. I continue to see him about his self-image and his means of coping.

Discussion

Christian Healing prayer can often lead to spontaneous healings, especially physical healings. In my experience, healing prayer in conjunction with medication, psychotherapy, and patient compliance (committed to making necessary changes) are often required for healing of one's illness, to discover the truth about self and God, and to have the ability to love, accept, and forgive one's self. It is typically an ongoing process.

There are now documented over 300 scientific meta analysis studies, 75% demonstrating conclusively that patients who have a faith belief in God fare much better in recovery from their illnesses, develop fewer complications, have a lower risk of serious illnesses, and actually live longer. This has been demonstrated in heart disease, cancer, surgery, mental illness, alcohol and drug abuse. Also the quality of family life is much better, and divorce rates are significantly lower.

It has been further demonstrated that those who attend church on a weekly basis and practice their religious beliefs experience even better health and recovery. Furthermore those who in addition to the above refrain from smoking and drinking alcohol, and exercise regularly, have the best prognosis.

Mental and emotional illness affects over one million Americans each year. Women are more affected than men.

1. Hertsgaard and Light (1984) of North Dakota State University in Fargo, found, in a study of 760 women, those with 2 or more children under age 14 years scored the highest for mental and emotional illness. However those who were churchgoers of at least once per month, and who were involved in the decision-making on the farm, had the lowest incidence.
2. In a 1990 study (Brown, Ndubuisi, & Gary) of 451 Afro-American men, there was a 2 time lower incidence of mental illness among regular churchgoers than among those who did not attend church.
3. A study in 1983 (Cook & Wimberley) examined coping with the deepest stress one could face, the loss of a loved one, especially a child. In 92 families with loss of a child, 70% found strength in religion. One year later 80% found strength in their faith and 40% actually felt stronger.

I see the benefits of Christian wholistic care to the patient as:
1. Development of a healthier lifestyle towards wholeness of body, mind and spirit;
2. Greater ability to help themselves manage their life's problems, through better self control and decision making;
3. Relationships with self, family, and others become more peaceful;
4. Patient's illness is healed or becomes more accepted and manageable;
5. Quality and fullness of life become more meaningful;
6. Increased productivity and less stress at work;
7. Reduced health costs;
8. Person becomes more of true authentic self.

I see the benefits to the physician/healthcare professional as:
1. Work becomes more enjoyable, fulfilling, and less stressful;

2. Relationships with patients become more compassionate, trusting, and respectful;
3. The risks of burnout, ligitation, and over work diminish;
4. Reduced office expenses, more peaceful office environment;
5. Personal spiritual growth in wholeness, holiness and new life;
6. Professional work and family life more balanced.

Bible References
1. Sirah 38 states that when you are sick, "first cleanse your heart." "Then seek the doctor, who will use herbs," and "will pray to the Lord that you may be healed."
2. Jn. 3:1. "His love is so great that we are called God's children."
3. I Thes. 5:23. "May the God who gives us peace, make you holy in every way and keep your whole being, spirit, mind and body, free from every fault, at the coming of Our Lord Jesus Christ."
4. Rom. 8:15-16. "God's Spirit joins himself to our spirit."
5. Rom. 8:5. "Those who live as the Spirit tells them to, have their minds controlled by what the Spirit wants."
6. Gal. 5:22-23. "The spirit produces love, joy, peace, patience, goodness, faithfulness, kindness, humility and self control."
7. Rom. 7:15. "We do not do the things we want to do but the things we hate."
8. Lk. 23:34. "Father forgive them, they do not know what they are doing."
9. Jn. 8:31-34. "You will know the truth and the truth will set you free, free from the sin that binds you and makes you a slave to your body."

Healing Prayer References
Kelsey, M. (1995). *Healing and Christianity: A Classic Study.* Minneapolis, MN: Augsburg Fortress Publishing.
Linn, M and Linn, D. (1988). *Healing Life's Hurts.* Mahwah, NJ: Paulist Press.
Linn, M., Ryan, B., and Linn, D. (1997). *To Heal as Jesus Healed.* Mineola, NY: Resurrection Press.
MacNutt, F. (1974). *Healing.* Notre Dame, IN: Ave Maria Press.
McAll, K. (1982). *Healing the Family Tree.* London: Sheldon Press.
Shlemon, B. (1982). *Healing the Hidden Self.* Notre Dame, IN: Ave Maria Press.

Medical Books and Journal References
Anderson, B.L., Kieclot-Glaser, J.K. and Glaser, R. (1994). "A behaviorial model of cancer stress and disease course." *American Psychologist, 49 (5):* 389-404.

Benson, H. and Stark, M. (1996). *Timeless Healing: The Power and Biology of Belief.* Collingdale, PA: Diane Publishing Co.

Bianchi, M., Sacerdote, P., Locatelli, L., Mantegazza, P. and Panerai, A. E. (1991). "Corticotropin releasing hormone, interleukin-1alpha, and tumor necrosis factor-alpha share characteristics of stress mediators." *Brain Research, 546(1)*: 139-142.

Breier, A., Albus, M., Pickar, D., Zahn, T.P., Wolkowitz, O.M. and Paul, S.M. (1987). "Controllable and uncontrollable stress in humans: Alterations in mood, neuroendrocine and psychophysiological function." *American Journal of Psychiatry, 144(11)*: 1419-1425.

Brown, D.R., Nduluisi, S.C. and Gary, L.E. (1990). "Religiosity and psychological distress among blacks." *Journal of Religion and Health, 29 (1):* 55-68.

Cacioppo, J.T., Malarkey, W.B., Kiecolt-Glaser, J.K., Uchino, B.N., Sqoutas-Emch, S.A., Sheridan, J.F., Bernstob, G.G. and Glaser, R. (1995). "Heterogeneity in neuroendocrine and immune responses to brief psychological stressors as a function of autonomic cardiac activation." *Psychosomatic Medicine, 57(2)*: 154-164.

Cook, J.A. and Wimberley, D.W. (1983). "If I should die before I wake: Religious commitment and adjustment to the death of a child." *Journal of the Scientific Study of Religion, 22(3):* 222-238.

Fulgosi, D. (2000). "Depression: The underlying cause of physical ailments." *Canadian Journal of Diagnosis*, 17(7): 82-93.

Gold, M.S. (1995). *The Good News About Depression: Cures and Treatments in the New Age of Psychiatry.* Westminster, PA: Bantam Books, Hormones, Ch. 9, p. 127.

Hamilton, S. (2001). "The bare bones on osteoporosis." *Canadian Journal of CME, 13(4):* 89-100.

House, A., Dennis, M., Mogridge, L., Hawton, K. and Warlow, C. (1990). "Life events and difficulties preceeding stroke." *Journal of Neurology, Neurosurgery and Psychiatry, 53(12)*: 1024-1028.

Hertsgaard, D. and Light, H. (1984). "Anxiety, depression and hostility in rural women." *Psychological Reports, 55(2):* 673-674.

Koenig, H, Mc Cullough, M.E. and Larson, D.B. (1998). *Handbook of Religion and Health.* Cary, NC: Oxford University Press, Part IV, pp. 231-357.

Koenig, H.G., Cohen, H.J., Blazer, D.G., Pieper, C., Meador, K.G., Shelp, F., Goli, V. and DiPasquale, B. (1992). "Religious coping and depression among elderly hospitalized medically ill men." *American Journal of Psychiatry 149(12):* 1693-1700.

Lehman, C.D., Rodin, J., McEwen, B. and Brinton, R. (1991). "Impact of environmental stress on the expression of insulin dependent disbetes melitus." *Behavorial Neurosci., 105(2)*: 241-245.

Levin, J.S. (1994). "Religion and health: Is there an association, is it valid, and is it causal?" *Social Science and Medicine* 38, (11): 1475-82.

Matthews, D. (1998). *The Faith Factor.* New York: Viking.

Mc Ewen, B.S. (1998). "Protective and damaging effects of stress mediators." *New England Journal of Medicine, 338*: 171-179.

Woolfrey, P. (2001). "The keys to figuring out Fibromyalgia." *Canadian Journal of CME, 13(4):* 71-85.

Key Words

Clinical-Spiritual-Medical terms were developed to help explain in a lay medical language some of the spiritual-clinical states as it relates to certain medical conditions.

1. *Broken Spirit* is the condition of a person's spirit that is partially or totally separated from the Spirit of God due to the effects of the spiritual legacy where the fundamental belief a person has of self and of God is false.
2. *Christian Spiritual Healing* is the process where the patient has freely chosen to invite the healing love of Jesus into his spirit through prayer, in order to forgive, to repent, to seek healing, and restoration to new life in accordance with God's will.
3. *Holiness* is a state of grace revealing the fruits of the Spirit: love, joy, peace, gentleness, kindness, faithfulness, and self control, in the perfection of charity and purity of heart (Gal 5:22).
4. *The Lie* is defined as the state of deception where the fundamental faith belief the patient has about self and about God is false but believes it to be true.
5. *New Life* is becoming one's true, authentic self to the fullest, with all one's unique gifts and talents.
6. *Religion* is the formal practice of your spiritual faith belief in God.
7. *The Secret* is the measures or means the patient takes to prove self as worthy, to gain acceptance, acknowledgement, or recognition, e.g. pleasing, perfectionism, seeking approval, workaholism, the joker, etc. It is based in the *lie*.
8. *Spirituality* is the experienced fundamental faith belief a person has acquired about his or her self, and God, in relation to their knowledge and lived experiences.
9. *Spiritual Legacy* is the patient's childhood lived experiences, where he or she might feel deprived of the affirming love necessary to become his or her true authentic self.
10. *Spiritual Stress* is a condition of mixed emotions of fear, guilt, and an-

ger, generated from feelings of being less than whole, defective, unloved, stupid, unworthy, not good enough, etc, due to the *broken spirit* and the *false belief*, the *lie* a person has about self.
11. The *whole person* is defined as a *spiritual human being*, made in the image and likeness of God.
12. *Wholeness* is the restoration of the patient's physical, emotional, mental, and psycho/social health and well being.

Chapter 3

Approaching Prayer in the Medical Setting

Thomas Newman M.D.
445 Elm St.
Denver, CO 80220

Practitioner

Thomas Newman, M.D., is a physician, certified in Internal Medicine. Following his graduation from the University of Colorado School of Medicine he received four years post graduate training at Presbyterian Hospital. His medical career included two years in the army, five years in private practice and his final twenty-six years in a large HMO in Denver, CO prior to his retirement in 1998. He is also a husband and father of three sons.

Journey of Integration

I previously detailed my conversion experience and receipt of the Baptism of the Holy Spirit which occurred in 1979 in the *Journal of Christian Healing* (Newman, 1991) as follows:

… I had an intellectual sort of spirituality - Sunday Mass, private prayer and a moral, ethical life. Later, my wife, Mary, and I would gather with friends and study various theological trends as expounded by Hans Küng and Pierre Teilhard de Chardin plus liberation and feminist theologians, and popular writings *demythologizing* the Scriptures. One night as we were driving home I quietly complained to God that I really didn't see much relevance in these theologies to my own daily living. Furthermore, I noted that the people of the early church must have had a different experience with him because the Scriptures said they were enthusiastic, joyful, and even willing to die for him. When I sat in front of the church looking at the people, I told him, I didn't see much happiness or joy, and I doubted that many of these would die for him. I doubted that I would either. Then I asked him: Was there some thing or some way in which he related to the early church that was different from what I experienced today - and would he please show me what it was?

About three months later, A close high school friend visited us. He turned the conversation to religion, then said, "If the Bible is the Word of God, what do you strip from it?" And then I heard within a voice say clearly: "Listen, this is what you have been looking for." For six hours, until 3 a.m., I listened with excitement as this friend opened the Scriptures to me. I drank with an unquenchable thirst. Although I declined prayer then for the Baptism of the Spirit, I spent several weeks reading Scripture and books on prayer and healing. I was dumbfounded. None of this related to my life's experiences. None of it was scientific. It was scriptural. Most compelling was that I heard a clear inner voice announcing the answer to my earlier, silent prayer.

Several weeks later, I sought prayer for the release of the gifts of the Holy Spirit in my life. I asked members of a traveling Protestant singing group that was visiting our local Catholic church to pray with me. Though nothing initially seemed to happen, later during the night as I prayed I began to laugh, and suddenly my laughter was overcome by prayer in tongues. I experienced an indescribable and overwhelming sense of being totally loved and totally forgiven. I felt totally cleansed before God. For more than six months I was on a high, and spent most of my free time in spontaneous prayer and praise. The responses to these prayers exploded my paradigm (p. 16-17).

Context

I also detailed in my previous article (Newman, 1991) several healings that occurred following prayer with some of my medical patients. I will briefly relate three of those healings plus some additional experiences to demonstrate my approach to prayer with patients in the medical setting.

Theory/Theology

Shortly after my conversion I read the book *How to Live Like a King's Kid* by Harold Hill and Irene Harrell (1974). The author, Harold Hill, an alcoholic, had been prayed with and was healed. He later prayed with an alcoholic friend who was also healed. Harold had asked his friend if he could compare his alcoholism to being in quicksand, sinking deeper with each try to get out. His friend said, "Yes, he could." Harold asked his friend to imagine himself in quicksand sinking, struggling, sinking deeper. Then he told his friend to notice someone approaching the edge of the quicksand, and then to realize that that someone was Jesus. "When you're ready," he told him, "ask Jesus to pull you out." The man did. He was healed as Harold had been before him.

Following Harold Hill's example I, then, prayed this prayer with two *hopeless* alcoholics, patients in my medical practice. The first, a woman, I prayed with by placing my hand upon her head and asking God, in silence, to help her in her need and to free her from alcoholism. The second, a man, I held while praying for God to love him through me and to meet him in his needs. I also asked God to not let anyone come into the room while I held the man. Both were healed the night we prayed. Both had craved alcohol throughout each day for years. Now neither had need of it. The woman became employed, was promoted, and generally blossomed. Her health improved but she refused counseling. The man experienced love as never before in his life and when taken to his hospital bed for detoxification felt like "A King's Kid" (his words not mine). He sought counseling and became a counselor. Both had always reacted to another's anger by grabbing a drink. The woman continued to do so, eventually lost her healing and returned to drinking. The man began to turn to drink again but his life flashed before him, he stopped, went to a hospital and stayed until his urge abated. He never drank again. I had prayed these prayers with them during a *window of opportunity*. In desperation both wanted freedom from alcoholism. Helpless, almost hopeless prayers had risen from their hearts as I prayed with them. Later I learned that a similar prayer led to the founding of AA and the Twelve-Step Program.

I was dumbfounded. I had witnessed God's Holy Spirit humbly answering a simple prayer with power, love, and peace. Realizing my church ignored and did not teach or preach about this kind of prayer for healing and that medicine rejected and disclaimed it, I joined the Association of Christian Therapists (ACT) to be with others practicing and experiencing this kind of prayer for healing. There I learned many aspects about praying with others. Two of these have been most helpful.

First, at the International ACT Conference in the Spring of 1981, Sr. Briege McKenna (1981) told of a vision she had received. In the vision Jesus showed her a tent and told her that she was the tent. Jesus came to live in that tent. At first she resisted but he told her that was where he lived so she let him in. He showed her that her problem was that she tried to be the one to meet all the needs of those who came to her for healing prayer. He informed her that they really came to see him and that if she would step aside and let him do the work he would do the healing.

Second, at the International ACT Conference in the Fall of 1981, Fr. Richard McAlear, O.M.I. (1981) speaking on *The Healing Power of the Cross*, related that all the experiences of the human heart were crystallized in the heart of Jesus. Where there was need for love, Jesus loved. Where there was need for mercy, Jesus had shown mercy. Where the human heart had been misunderstood, Jesus had also been misunderstood. Where there was rejection, Jesus had been rejected, even by those close to him. When there was betrayal, Jesus had been betrayed. When words had been twisted, so were his. Where there had been humiliation, Jesus too had been humiliated, even being stripped naked in public for others to see. Where there has been mockery, so Jesus was mocked. Jesus was deserted by friends and even felt deserted by God. Jesus suffered anguish so great that he shed tears of blood. Jesus was led away, bound out of his control. Jesus was brutalized, tortured and murdered. Jesus loved and forgave. Jesus sought quiet prayer, and he enjoyed the company of others. Jesus lived in poverty. Jesus knew the grieving of death in his family and friends. Jesus also understood and knew the healing power of God.

Methodology

When persons come to a physician, a therapist, a nurse etc., they come to a healer. In our society our degrees, training, scientific skills and *stethoscope* are outward signs of being a healer. We listen, examine, diagnose and then treat to the limits of our skills and science. We acknowledge these limits. But looking beyond this apparent reality to a greater reality, we see that the patient has come to the tent of the healer who dwells inside.

I approach praying with a patient by asking the patient if he or she would like to pray a prayer together in silence. I pray silently to get out of Jesus' way. I tell the patient that Jesus understands, that in his heart he has experienced what they are feeling or going through. I ask them to picture Jesus and tell him what is on their heart, how they feel, what they request of him - whatever comes to mind. I intercede while they are doing this, pleading with Jesus to pour out his love on that person and respond to their need, all in silence. I usually rest my hand on a hand or shoulder rarely, but occasionally, on the person's head.

Case Illustrations
Case 1

A patient I previously reported (Newman, 1991, p. 19-20), I will again detail here. This woman came to me in a panic. Her psychotherapist called informing me that the patient was panicking and that she was sexually abused in childhood. She had been in therapy for twelve years with little or no progress. She arrived in panic. The examining room was small. She was constantly moving about. She got on the table, off the table, sat, stood, walked, talked, respiration increasing - all of this faster and faster, and all the while demanding I do something to help her. I offered psychiatric help. She refused. I offered medication. She refused. Her demands accelerated. The tempo of her hyperactivity continued to crescendo. About forty minutes passed, nothing was gained. Five o'clock approached and those in the mental health department would be leaving. I was beginning to catch her contagious panic. She was terrified that because she had been abused as a child she would become an abusive parent though she never abused or had thoughts of abusing her children.

She told me that when she was growing up, her father, brothers and she had played strip poker. She always lost. Her father and brothers would mock and tease her. Following that, her father took her to the bedroom where he further abused her. She now panicked at the thought she could become an abuser. She wanted help. She had refused what I could offer as a physician. I could do nothing medically, so I asked if she would be willing to pray with me and see if God would help us find a way to help her. As a child she once attended a Pentecostal service, taken to it by those who had abused her. But she was willing to pray.

I told her that Jesus understood. I told her that Jesus had been stripped naked in public and was humiliated by those around him. I asked her to picture Jesus and tell him how she felt. She could do it silently and I would pray quietly. A few minutes passed and she began to sob - deep sobs. Gradually her breathing slowed, her sobs softened and abated, tears flowed freely. Quietly she looked at me. From deep within she experienced relief. She burst out with tears still flowing, "He understood. It's the first time anyone has understood. He understands." She then said, "This is the first time I have been able to cry about this. Thank you." This woman had come to seek the healer. Somehow the eyes of her soul saw beyond the training and the stethoscope, beyond the door of the tent to the Healer residing inside. She had dismissed my medical offerings and had demanded the Healer do something. When she met him and pleaded her cause, he let her know he understood and graced her with his love, mercy and peace.

She would now accept medications and a referral to one of our psychiatrists. Later she began having a memory that again caused panic. She remembered going out on an isolated dirt road with her father, getting out of the vehicle and walking a distance. At the point she could remember no further, she became filled with fear. She called, I told her to come in. I asked her to picture Jesus with her on that road and tell him what she felt. I prayed silently. Soon she was again at peace, looked up and said, "He knew I said, 'No'." Her panic and fear ceased for then. That was the last time I saw her.

Case 2

Praying in tongues when we do not know how to pray or what to pray for, is another way that I pray. However, in a medical setting, this might seem a bit unusual. One day in prayer I asked God if praying in tongues silently counts? It was one of those questions I posed to him from time to time never sure if I would get an answer.

One wintry evening as I was about to finish my day a nurse told me that one of Dr. Tim's patients had just walked in. Dr. Tim and the other physicians had gone home. I was tired and did not want to see another patient after I completed the one I was about to see. The nurse went on to say that the person was living in his van and had been vomiting all day. I was suddenly aware in my *knower* that God had sent this patient to me. The weather was getting worse and a van was no place to stay. Perhaps I was to medicate him and put him up somewhere. I said I would see him. Sal was sitting on the examining table unable to lie down because that caused severe vertigo and vomiting. He was becoming dehydrated. I decided to admit him to the hospital overnight and re-hydrate him. The next morning, armed with his chart held palm up in my right hand, I went to see Sal who had been sitting up all night lest he vomit. I tried to slowly roll the head of his bed down but he sat bolt upright and leaning over the edge of the bed began dry heaves. I remembered my childhood and how good it felt to have my head held while vomiting, so left palm up I held his forehead. Both palms now up, I recognized a position of prayer. I began to pray in tongues silently, mouth closed, no lip motion. He concluded his episode, sat up and looked at me saying, "Were you praying?" "Yes," I replied. He asked me to pray again with him. We prayed the *Our Father*. I then changed the subject and examined him. We would be running further tests and he would be staying another day. The next day I went to see him and he asked, "When you were praying with me yesterday, were you praying in the Spirit?" "Yes," I replied somewhat taken back. I promptly changed the subject, addressed his medical problems telling him we needed further testing and consultation. As I entered his room the following morning he asked, "Do you want to know how I knew you were praying in the Spirit?" "Yes, how did you?" I asked. He responded, "The moment you started to pray, I felt the power." I had nothing I could say. I thanked him for telling me, addressed his medical issues and left. God had answered my question. But that was only part of why God sent Sal who was now developing a number of neurological changes in his initial acute episode of multiple sclerosis. Sal witnessed to and prayed with a number of physicians and nurses. While he prayed with a patient advocate, she received the gift of praying in tongues. It would be six months before I had the courage to ask what he meant when he said he "felt the power." He told me that as I began to pray, he felt the love of God and an awareness that God had placed him where he was, surrounded by those God wanted around him and that he was not to fear. Several months later, Sal drove a wheelchair bound man 800 miles to a healing service in Texas. A helper came to Sal telling him to come forward to the stage. As he started to bring the man in the wheelchair, the helper said that it was Sal the Lord wished to heal. Upon his return, all abnormal neurological findings had disappeared. Sal then moved away.

Case 3

At times, prayer to bring peace and consolation seem most appropriate. Then I may speak aloud briefly, asking God to bring his peace and love and be palpably present to that person. Then I pray silently. In part, this approach dissipates the person's foreboding that the doctor is going to pray a little theology or sermon over a person. However, the greater reason is to step out of the way of the Healer in the tent.

Karen, legally blind, on kidney dialysis three times weekly for several years, had painful diabetic neuropathy, frequent and severe angina and persistent itching from extensive psoriasis and renal failure. She had spoken to her nephrologist about discontinuing dialysis but first there was a wedding, a graduation and an anniversary. When she discussed her tentative decision with me, she had grown weary beyond her endurance of chronic pain, severe fatigue and the effort required to be tethered to a machine three of every seven days. Her husband who loved her and didn't want to lose her suffered in her suffering. Though she asked what I thought, she was seeking my support of her decision. I inquired about her prayer life and then asked if she would like to pray to invite God to help direct us. Initially she was hesitant. Then she agreed when I told her we would each pray silently. Several weeks later she was hospitalized with pneumonia and as I was discharging her, her husband came and called me aside. As he started to speak he broke down crying, thanking me for praying with his wife. He looked at me saying, "You'll never understand, there is no way you could understand how much your praying with my wife that day in the office meant to both of us." About a month later she called to tell me she had discontinued dialysis. I visited her at home and after reminiscing good times, she, her husband, her sister and I prayed together and hugged our final good-bye.

Case 4

Sometimes God simply wants to reach someone through us.

An elderly man and woman moved to Denver to be with their remaining son. They came to me and related that six months earlier their younger son, who had been their emotional and often physical support, died in his sleep of a myocardial infarction leaving a wife and two children. The woman was a believing Christian. The man was agnostic. Neither had graced a church for years. The woman was passing through normal grief. The man's grief was accompanied with moderately severe depression though he was not suicidal at the time. He refused medications or psychiatric help. He did not believe in that. He told me he was not like me or his wife. He did not believe in psychiatrists or God though he wished he could. Several days later he returned, now suicidal. He laid out his life and wept. He agreed to accept medication and see a psychiatrist. I was about to leave the room when he once again said, "I wish I could believe like you and my wife but I just don't." I asked, "Would you be willing to pray together and ask that 'if God, you really do exist, will you let me know some way'?" "Yes." We prayed in silence asking God to show him and help him. I wrote a prescription and arranged for the urgent psychiatric appointment. The next day the nurse brought me a note requesting I call the patient ASAP. "It's important, but don't worry." Instantly I knew God had touched him, perhaps healed him. While watching television the evening before, he suddenly experienced peace, his depression lifted, he could think clearly (this had been difficult for several years because of an underlying depression), he had joy and he knew that God had touched him. He returned to let me know he was all right and no longer depressed. Several months later he and his wife returned to their former city to help his daughter-in-law with her children. He would weep when he recalled the night Jesus touched him. He now prayed and read the Bible regularly with his wife. He said, "I now know the reason we moved to Denver was not to be with our son, but to see you." I reminded him it was God and not me that had done the healing. "Yes, but God wanted us to see you to accomplish that."

Discussion

These were situations in which I had no control except to offer to pray with the patient. The patient prayed from the heart after hitting bottom. I interceded reminding Jesus that this was his child, I could do nothing, it was over my head, please meet the patient with your love. I am certain now, that whenever I pray with a patient or someone else for healing, God is listening, pressing his ear to our lips. I also know God will respond every time in love for that person. I know God desires an intimate and personal relationship with each of us. I am now able to pray with complete confidence that God will respond to the need of the person with love. I believe that God prepares the heart, and that the time for this prayer is when the heart of the person is ready to call upon God. Sirach 38:1–15 tells us that when we become ill we ought first to pray then seek the physician who, when applying his or her skills, continues in the creative work of God. The vision of the tent helps me understand this Scripture and approaching prayer in the medical setting.

References

Hill, H. and Harrell, I. (1974). *How to Live Like a King's Kid*. Plainfield, NJ: Logos Associates.

McAlear, R. (1981). *The Healing Power of the Cross*. One audio tape is available by contacting: Robin Caccese, 137 Proudfoot Drive, Birdsboro, PA 19508, Phone: (610) 582-5571; email: rcaccese@talon.net.

McKenna, B. (1981). Testimony and Praying for Cancer Patients. Two audio tapes are available by contacting: Robin Caccese, 137 Proudfoot Drive, Birdsboro, PA 19508, Phone: (610) 582-5571; email: rcaccese@talon.net.

Newman, T. (1991). "Resolving the physician's conflict between two worlds." *Journal of Christian Healing, 13*:1, 14-22.

Chapter 4

Integrating Medical, Psychotherapeutic and Prayer Modalities: A Case Study*

Len Sperry, M.D., Ph.D.
Barry University
11300 NE Second Avenue
Miami Shores, FL 33161

Practitioner

Len Sperry, M.D., Ph.D. is Clinical Professor of Psychiatry and Behavioral Medicine at the Medical College of Wisconsin and also Professor at Barry University, Miami Shores, FL. He is board certified in Psychiatry, Preventive Medicine and Clinical Psychology, is a Fellow of the American Psychiatric Association, the American College of Preventive Medicine, and the Division of Psychology and Religion of the American Psychological Association, as well as a member of the Committee on Psychiatry and Religion of the Group for the Advancement of Psychiatry (GAP). He is listed in *Best Doctors in America,* 1999 - 2000.

Journey of Integration

My first exposure to healing prayer was Francis MacNutt and Agnes Sanford at *Camp Farthest Out* in San Diego in the summer of 1975. I read and re-read MacNutt's book, *Healing* (1974). Soon afterwards Father Jerry Bevalaqua, O.S.A. invited me to join his healing team, and by fall I began incorporating healing prayer into my professional practice. I joined ACT in the fall of 1975 and began attending ACT conferences in the spring of 1976 where I learned much about other forms of healing prayer such as soaking prayer and experienced deep personal healing. These experiences expanded my appreciation of medical psychotherapy and psychiatry as a biopsychosocial approach to that of a integrated biopsychosociospiritual approach.

Context

The context of this illustration is an outpatient medical and psychotherapy practice setting. T. is a 33 year old divorced male referred by a Catholic couple who were concerned about the traditional medical care that T. had been receiving. This couple was active in the Charismatic Renewal and had some experience with the healing prayer ministry.

---

* First published in the *Journal of Christian Healing*, Volume 22, Number 1&2, Spring/Summer, 2000, pp. 44-50.

Goal

The initial goal of treatment was to stabilize and detoxify this rather ill patient, increase his immunocompetence and analyze his fear of rejection and abandonment. Rather soon the goal expanded to focus more on the spiritual factors that appeared to exacerbate his medical symptoms, including his image of God.

Theory/Theology: Soaking Prayer

A biopsychosociospiritual understanding of personhood was central in formulating this case. Unlike physically healthy individuals who present for psychotherapy, spiritual direction or inner healing prayer, individuals like T. come to treatment with wounding that is pervasive in their body, mind and spirit, and often within their social support system. While sometimes the Lord may instantly effect a healing and a cure in such a seriously ill or injured individual, this is the exception rather than the norm. More often, healing tends to follow a incremental process, particularly when psychic trauma has been severe and chronic. Such pervasive wounding usually requires a integrative, multi-modal approach rather than a single treatment modality. Soaking prayer was one of several modalities utilized in this case. Since, I believe soaking prayer played such a key role in this case, and because it is a relatively unknown form of healing prayer, it will be briefly described.

According to MacNutt, the term *soaking prayer* is attributed to the Reverend Tommy Tyson, a major figure in the healing ministry in America. MacNutt describes this form of prayer: "Soaking prayer conveys the idea of time to let something seep through to the core of something dry that needs to be revived. That's the way it is with the laying on of hands when we feel that God is asking us to irradiate the sickness with his power and love" (MacNutt, 1977, p. 39). In the early days of his healing ministry, MacNutt found that individuals with chronic illnesses, like arthritis, who were initially prayed for with the laying on of hands might experience a small improvement such as a slight reduction in pain or small increase in joint mobility. He found that in individuals where "some healing had already started to take place, then further prayer would usually lead to still more healing. As a crude example: if about 10 percent of a healing had already started to take place through the first prayer, then, after praying for another 40 minutes, there might be something like a 50 percent improvement" (p.41). MacNutt cites a number of parables which involve the injunction to "pray without ceasing" to offer support for the practice of soaking prayer.

More recently, soaking prayer was the basic treatment modality in a prospective study conducted by Dale Matthews, M.D. Matthews collaborated with MacNutt and prayer teams from the MacNutt's *Christian Healing Ministries* in the first prospective clinical trial of this form of prayer. Called the

Clearwater Rheumatoid Arthritis Study, Matthews' study was designed to test the effects of healing prayer on study subjects with chronic rheumatoid arthritis. This prayer study protocol included several sessions each day of *soaking prayer*, or intensive, hour-long periods of laying on of hands and prayer by two prayer ministers with each patient as well as teaching sessions about the nature of spiritual healing (Matthews, 1998, p. 77). Preliminary results of this study (Matthews, Marlowe, MacNutt, 2000) suggest that those receiving soaking prayer showed statistically significant differences, as well as significant (substantial) clinical improvement compared to control subjects. Furthermore, a follow up after the study was completed showed that most maintained their improved health status. For a chronic illness that heretofore was believed to be manageable but not curable, the study results seem to many to be incredible. As a result of the experience of his prayer ministry teams, MacNutt changed the healing prayer protocol at the *Christian Healing Ministries'* Center in Jacksonville, Florida to a soaking prayer format. In short, soaking prayer is an intensive, ongoing form of healing prayer that has been found most effective when traditional, single occasion prayer for physical or mental healing appears to have a limited response.

As the following case history will illustrate, prior experiences of occasional healing prayer seemingly effect no observable change in a deeply wounded individual with significant medical illness. However, a combination of one-on-one prayer along with soaking prayer and integrated with medical and psychotherapeutic modalities may and often does effect major changes, including a cure, as illustrated with this case.

Methodology

To conceptualize a complex case, particularly with a chronic medical and/or psychiatric presentation, a biopsychosociospiritual perspective (Sperry, 1986) is helpful. This requires a biopsychosociospiritual assessment which is the basis for developing an integrative, multimodal treatment plan. Such an assessment is comprehensive, and in the spiritual domain, usually involves understanding the individual's early bonding and attachment to love objects, capacity for self-transcendence, and image of God. Chronic illnesses that are seemingly unresponsive to traditional and alternative medical treatment or even to ongoing healing prayer may be an indication that the basic or original trauma was prenatal or perinatal, as this case seems to suggest.

Case Illustration

T. presented with symptoms of fatigue, anorexia, hypersomnia, low energy and decreased motivation. Besides a yellowish-green tinge to his skin, he appeared to be lifeless and emaciated. He reported a 28 lb. weight loss over the past 4 months. He denied that he was depressed or suicidal. T. was a teacher but had been on a medical leave of absence for some six weeks prior to our first contact. He previously had been diagnosed by three internists with chronic hepatitis, and indicated that he had experienced four episodes of intense exacerbations of symptoms lasting from 6-18 months since the age of 18. The last episode being two years previously. He had been divorced approximately two years earlier, and had experienced considerable loneliness and was without much of a social support network, except for an older married couple. The couple was health-conscious and were concerned that the traditional medical treatment that T. was receiving, including corticosteroid injections weekly, were not helping. Although never having met me, they encouraged T. to consult with me. I began by performing a complete biopsychosociospiritual assessment.

Besides chronic active hepatitis (most likely non-A, non-B type), T. had a history of asthma and chronic sinusitis and apparently was sufficiently immunocompromised that he contracted upper respiratory infections on the average of 5 to 6 times a year, sometimes resulting in hospitalization for the treatment of bronchial pneumonia. There was positive family history of heart disease, lung cancer and depression. Despite his denial of depression, T. reported five episodes of untreated depression since the age of 15. Three of the episodes preceded exacerbation of chronic hepatitis and all were triggered by a significant interpersonal rejection.

The developmental history indicated that T. was the older of two children. He has a younger brother, Jack, who was a basketball star in high school and college and is now a successful corporate attorney who is rarely ill. His brother has been the father's favorite since his birth. T. recalls feeling unwanted and abandoned as a child. His mother had once confided to T. that his father had dreamed of having sons who were highly successful athletes and businessmen. From the moment T. was born, by cesarean section, he was sickly and disappointed his father greatly. Reportedly, the father spent little time with T. and instead doted on Jack. While his mother did spend time with T, it seemed to involve taking him to doctor appointments and lab tests for his seemingly constant medical conditions.

Spiritually, T struggled with faith and hope although he continued to be a practicing Catholic. His image of God was harsh, demanding and distant. His prayer life was uneven, particularly when he was experiencing symptomatic exacerbations. He was reasonably active in a Charismatic prayer community and while he had availed himself of the healing prayer ministry on a few occasions in the past four months, he noted no observable changes.

Laboratory tests confirmed the presence of chronic hepatitis (antibodies to non-A, non-B hepatitis agent, the immunoglobulin M (IgM) antibody, and elevated hepatic enzymes AST and ALT). My first concern was to gradually wean the steroids and build up his immunocompetence. Within four weeks he was completely weaned from the steroids.

At the same time I began him on a regimen of natural remedies including liver and thyroid abstracts, and prescribed a detoxification diet regimen. Healing prayer was a brief part of our weekly medical psychotherapy sessions. In my morning prayers I would regularly pray for individual patients and would ask the Lord for discernment and guidance on diagnostic and treatment issues. In prayer the morning after I had seen T. for the second time, I sensed that soaking prayer (MacNutt, 1977) was indicated as an adjunct to my weekly sessions with him. I also got an image of T. being prayed over in front of the Eucharist by an older couple. When I mentioned this to T. at our third appointment, he immediately noted that his friends - the older couple - had just offered to pray over him every morning after the Eucharistic prayer service at their church. They had suggested that T. ask my opinion of such a plan. Since T. had been skeptical of healing prayer because of his prior experience, soaking prayer was described along with its indications and applications, particularly with chronic illness. I reviewed what I had learned about soaking prayer from Francis MacNutt and gave T. a paper about it for him to read. Although he was feeling and looking better - his yellowish-green tinged skin was fading - probably because of the detoxification diet and supplements - he became noticeably pale as he expressed his fear and ambivalence about the couple's offer. He was uncertain about the daily time commitment and *being a burden* to the couple. I was able to clarify and then interpret his resistance noting that since he had felt unwanted and abandoned as a child he could not conceive of anyone wanting to spend hours a week nurturing him with prayer. T. was taken back by this interpretation and left saying he would think and pray about it.

The next time I saw T., he was beaming as he introduced the older couple to me. They expressed their commitment to begin praying with T. They had never engaged in this prayer form, although they had been to a healing where it had been described and demonstrated. So, soaking prayer became part of an integrated treatment plan consisting of medical treatment - particularly involving detoxification measures such as fruit fasts and botanical enemas, as well as a therapeutic diet and nutritional supplements - spiritually-oriented psychotherapy, and healing prayer in my office. It was mutually agreed that the soaking prayer would occur 5-6 days a week for 30-45 minutes following reception of the Eucharist by all three, and that the prayer would occur in the presence of the Holy Eucharist. Since this couple functioned as sacristans at their church, they were confident that their pastor would endorse this activity.

This integrated treatment continued for approximately three months. It seemed to me that the soaking prayer seemed to *supercharge* the combined medical and psychotherapeutic treatment. By that time, T. had regained his energy level, weight and motivation. His skin was now clear and he had been without any respiratory symptoms for some 10 weeks, a record for him. He had returned to his school in the past week where he functioned as a substitute teacher since it was nearly the end of the school year. This return to work had necessitated a change in the soaking prayer to weekends. After two weeks it was stopped by mutual decision. Our therapy, however, continued for another four months during which we focused largely on inner healing themes including his relationship with his parents, his feelings of being abandoned and unwanted, and his image of God. By the seventh month his image of God was becoming less harsh and more nurturing and accepting. At eleven months, sessions were shifted to a biweekly schedule as we began to enter the termination phase. At fourteen months we mutually agreed to a meet on a quarterly basis to follow his medical and psychotherapeutic progress. Approximately, eighteen months after we began treatment, lab testing showed no markers of any liver damage, something that the medical textbooks cannot explain.

Discussion

One possible explanation of these lab test findings is that T. had been completely healed of chronic hepatitis by the combination of treatment, including healing prayer. Another possible explanation is that there was a laboratory error. To rule this possibility out, I contacted the lab about rerunning the serological tests. The results were the same. So, it seemed reasonable to conclude that T. was both healed and cured. Since I believe that grace builds on nature, I suspect it is not unreasonable to assume that the various medical and psychotherapeutic modalities worked synergistically with the healing prayer, particularly the soaking prayer in the context of a loving a supportive Christian community.

References

MacNutt, F.(1974). *Healing.* Notre Dame, IN: Ave Marie Press.

MacNutt, F.(1977). *The Power to Heal.* Notre Dame, IN: Ave Marie Press.

Matthews, D. (1998). *The Faith Factor: Proof of the Healing Power of Prayer.* New York: Viking.

Matthews, D.A., Marlowe, S.M. and MacNutt, F.S. (2000). "Effects of intercessory prayer on patients with Rheumatoid Arthritis." *Southern Medical Journal, 92(12):* 1177-1186.

Sperry, L. (1986). "Care of body, care of spirit: Dimensions of spiritual well-being." *Journal of Christian Healing,* 8:2, 27-31.

Nursing Practice

Chapter 5

Parish Nursing in Another Faith Tradition*

Bernice M. DeBoer, R.N., B.S.N., Parish Nurse
N77W15955 Hunters Ridge Circle.
Menomonee, WI 53051

Practitioner

Bernice M. DeBoer, R.N., B.S.N., Parish Nurse, completed formal parish nurse education through the Parish Nurse Institute of Marquette University in 1995. She is actively involved in planning and implementing the Elmbrook Parish Nurse Program, the first formally designated parish nurse program within the Covenant system. She presented the proposal for the initiation of the Parish Nurse Program sponsored by St. Joseph's Hospital of Milwaukee, WI and assisted with developing that program. Bernice also serves as an active member of the Covenant Health Care System Pastoral Care Re-Design Team and the Milwaukee Archdiocesan Parish Nurse/Health Ministry Task force. She plans to expand her own parish nurse ministry to two additional congregations.

Context

For me parish nursing is ecumenical. I am Roman Catholic by faith tradition and practice. Yet I carry out a parish nursing ministry in a Lutheran parish affiliated with the Evangelical Lutheran Church of America (ELCA). The hospital that sponsors me, Elmbrook Memorial Hospital, is part of a group out of Wheaton Franciscan Services within the Covenant Healthcare System of Wisconsin. This is an ecumenical expression of their mission to human and community development and to serve those in need.

Case Illustration

My practice and ministry to members of Christ the King Lutheran congregation in Brookfield, Wisconsin, encompasses all of the traditional roles integral to the practice of parish nursing in most settings. In this article I will illustrate some aspects of my personal experience specific to my work in this parish.

Christ the King supports several members specially trained as *Stephen Ministers*. *Stephen Ministry* is an ecumenical program that equips lay people

---

* First published in *The Journal of Christian Healing*, Volume 18, Number 4, Winter, 1996, pp. 19-21.

to provide one-on-one support to individuals experiencing need and loss. A particular part of this program focuses upon teaching effective listening and responding skills within a confidential environment. When issues surface that require resources beyond their scope the Stephen Ministers actively seek out sources to help resolve those problems. Stephen Ministries is essentially the Health Ministry team for this congregation. I work closely with them to listen and to access resources and make referrals for health and mental health care. Other times, I become the *Stephen Minister* to the Stephen Minister as they individually come to me with issues of their own. In addition I am in the process of "tapping" their talents and expertise to collaborate with our youth director in presenting a program to teach the high-school students appropriate peer listening and responding skills. Indirectly, this activity may be a positive force to bridge communication between different generations.

Christ the King hosts a pre-school program for three and four year olds. This has also become a context of ministry for me. I have, for most of my professional career, practiced in a predominantly adult world and have used adult language and frames of reference. It has become no small feat for me to transfer teaching content from an adult perception to a pre-school context. I literally thank God that there are gifted resource persons who can assume the mind of the child and willingly share this knowledge with me. I will soon be presenting a program to pre-schoolers about the more common medical equipment these youngsters may encounter in their experience of health care.

Frequently parish nurses minister to a member of the Church's pastoral team. (I have permission to use the following story from Pastor Grindeland.) For almost a year, Pastor Gary Grindeland of Christ the King, age 43, experienced serious health problems himself. At Thanksgiving, 1995 he underwent a craniotomy for an intracerebral venous bleed that originated from an arterio-venous malformation. He returned to active ministry in February, 1996 and functioned quite well until July, 1996 when he began experiencing severe vertigo and visual disturbances. It was eventually thought, after much evaluation, that these symptoms were related to a CVA (Cardio Vascular Accident) somewhere in the brainstem. As a parish nurse, I have and continue to accompany Pastor Gary through recovery from these events by listening, counseling and support activities. I helped him plan for his return to active ministry on a limited schedule in January, 1997. Part of this planning work dealt with establishing a time schedule for his being on site and deciding what activities he was up to doing, for example, planning for him to either celebrate liturgy or preach, but not to do both at once.

Out of the preceding events and experiences came the introduction of a ritual new to this congregation but a valid part of Lutheran tradition, that of a service of healing and anointing. As an extension of a round the clock prayer vigil for Pastor Gary and his family, the interim pastor and I proposed doing an anointing service for him. Pastor Gary was very receptive to this. This service was done within the context of Sunday morning worship. For me personally, a most powerful moment came when the celebrant asked me, after he laid on hands, to perform the actual anointing with oil. This was a visible sign of what Pastor Gary believes to be the wholistic connection, that demonstrable sign of how our physical and psycho-emotional natures are intimately bound up with our spiritual selves. This was a manifestation of the Gospel mandate "to heal." As an outgrowth of this experience, we offered this same ritual to members of the congregation at three other worship services the following month. About 25 members chose to receive anointing. I anticipate that we will repeat this service at intervals from now on.

Parish nursing is also outreach. It goes beyond the boundaries of actual church membership. Recently, the interim pastor, Ed Ruen, the Social Ministry Committee, and I collaborated together to bring a presentation about "Forgiveness as Healing" by Prof. Robert Enright of the University of Wisconsin-Madison to Christ The King parish. The community at large was invited and approximately 175 people came out on a cold winter evening to hear about forgiveness. A positive piece of that experience related to the communication and community-building that took place after the formal program. There was so much communication still occurring that at 10 P.M. we had to announce that we were closing the doors to the church for the night.

Discussion

In relating my experiences as parish nurse at Christ The King Lutheran Church, I have attempted to describe the real life situations and contexts through which the whole ministry has manifested. Parish nursing is about connecting with self, with individuals, with groups, with community, and, maybe, even with all of God's creation. It is a powerful instrument for "bridge-building" wherever its sphere of influence extends and is felt.

Chapter 6

Healing the Dying*

Sister Mary Jane Linn, C.S.J., R.N.
Matthew Linn, S.J.
Dennis Linn, S.J.
Re-Member Ministries
3914-A Michigan Ave.
St. Louis, MO 63118

Practitioners

Sister Mary Jane Linn, C.S.J. was a registered nurse who held a master's degree in nursing education from the Catholic University of America and a post-masters degree in psychiatric mental health nursing from the University of California, Berkeley. For over twenty years, Sister taught in and was chairman of the Department of Nursing at the College of St. Catherine, St. Paul, Minnesota.

In the years before her death, Sister Mary Jane received permission from her religious community, the Sisters of St. Joseph of Carondelet, to spend her full time in praying for the ministry of her cousins Matthew and Dennis Linn. Sister frequently joined her cousins in giving retreats and workshops. When she was at home, she gave directed retreats and assisted in the pastoral care of the members of her religious community in retirement at Bethany Convent in St. Paul, Minnesota.

Sister Mary Jane died on June 2, 1979, shortly after completing the manuscript for the book *Healing the Dying* with Matthew and Dennis Linn. The book's theme is: a person can complete their unfinished business in life and can then choose death. Her cousin Dennis wrote in the preface to *Healing the Dying*, "Once she wrote her book, she had completed her unfinished business and I think chose to die (p.ix)."

Matthew and Dennis Linn have spent many years conducting healing workshops for such diverse groups as religious communities, ecumenical congregations and medical personnel in many countries. Besides having worked as hospital chaplains and psychotherapists at Wohl Psychiatric Clinic, they have taught courses on healing at Marquette University, at the Universidad Ibero Americana in Mexico City, and an American Medical Association course to doctors. They have published a total of 17 books, many

---

* Excerpts from *Healing the Dying* by Mary Jane Linn, CSJ; Matthew Linn, S.J.; Dennis Linn, S.J.; copyright by The Missionary Society of St. Paul the Apostle in the State of New York. Used with permission of Paulist Press. www.paulistpress.com

with Sheila Fabricant Linn. These books speak of ways of praying which bring physical, psychological and spiritual wholeness.

Context
   The retirement community of the Sisters of St. Joseph of Carondelet, Bethany Convent, St. Paul, MN.

Goal
   To assist in the pastoral care of the members of her religious community in retirement.

Case Illustrations
Case One
Father, forgive them, they know not what they do (Luke 23:34).
   "Rita," I whispered, putting my hand in hers, "I came to be with you."
   "Come, be with me. Get them to pray," she begged.
   Her begging eyes confirmed what we both knew in our hearts: Rita was about to die. We had spoken of it together many times before. However, none of the others across the hall from her believed that she would die this time anymore than all the other times when she had had a "bad spell." For some years, she told me, she (now 82) had been wearing a pacemaker to regulate her heartbeat, and frequently when she became careless or when something went amiss with the pacemaker it would seem to her and to those very close to her that she would surely die. But often by the next day she would be up and around making sure that everyone knew she was still alive. As this happened again and again, people around her were inclined not to believe her - this, she told me, hurt her.
   But this time there would be no next day. Her plea, "Get them to pray," had come from deep within her. She seemed to feel that now it really was her turn to go to God, to reach at last her eternal reward. She wanted her sisters to pray for her now, as she had done so often for those who had gone before her. She had helped me a lot. Just a few days before she had been the one to organize the deathwatch for a dying friend. "How shall we pray?" she had asked. We stopped for a moment to ask Jesus how he wanted us to pray, then Rita began her task of soliciting prayers for the person. She was good, too, at encouraging others by her words, "Pray longer until the end comes."
   Now, as I went from person to person asking prayers for her, I was struck by the fact that not one person was ready to do the same for her; no one really believed that she was, indeed, on her deathbed. The response I got from almost everyone to whom I spoke was, "Wait and see, she'll be up and around tomorrow. You've been here for only a couple of months. You just don't realize yet how she always comes back to life."

So it happened that no one intented to go with me to be with Rita. No one. It saddened me. And I knew it saddened Rita. When I returned, she said bitterly, "They don't believe you, do they?" I saw a tear run down her left cheek as I knelt down.

Kneeling beside her I wondered how to pray for her. I began to pray in my heart, "Lord, have mercy on us in our blindness, and hardness of heart. Father, forgive us ...."

"Stay," she begged, "I want to die this time." Then I understood with unquestionable clarity that my prayer for her was simply to be with her, interceding with the Father, in the name of Jesus,[1] for the gift of forgiveness and love until Jesus himself would come for her.

"Rita," I whispered softly, "until Jesus comes for you, I will stay. I will pray as he leads me to pray for you; all you need to do is rest in the arms of our Father. I will do the praying. If you want anything, I will be here. I will remain until he comes to take you to heaven."

I signed Rita's forehead and hands with blessed oil[2] - earlier that day she had received sacramental anointing. Sitting beside her, I put my hand on hers and began to pray gently: "Lord Jesus, thank you for your love for Rita. I ask that in your mercy you give her the gift to love and forgive her sisters. I know, as you know, Lord, that if they really understood Rita's condition, they, too, would be interceding for her now. I ask you, Jesus, to replace any darkness in and around Rita with your light and life. Thank you, Jesus." I continued to pray as I was led and was soon joined by the mother superior of the Bethany sisters.

By supper time some of the sisters finally became aware of the seriousness of Rita's condition. They had seen us praying with her and one after another they stopped and, from where they were in the doorway, joined in prayer. One friend stood at the bedside for a long time and held her hand. Although Rita was struggling to catch her breath she managed to whisper, "Thank you." The next few hours were gentle, quiet.

A little after midnight she raised herself up on her elbows and murmured, "You are still here .... Tell them I forgive .... I do not blame them .... Father, forgive them .... Stay," and then she collapsed.

As Rita slipped into unconsciousness, I realized that at just this moment she had let go of life, that this time it was possible for her to die because our being with her had made it possible for her to forgive.

I stayed. She died at 6:45 in the morning. Would Rita have died, I wonder, any of those other times had she, like Jesus, reached the moment of forgiveness?

Father, forgive them, they know not what they do.

Case Two
My God, my God, why have you forsaken me? (Matthew 27:46)
When he was dying, Jesus anguished and his anguish had to be heard. So it was with Lucy, who, it seems to me, anguished more than any of the others; and it was she with whom I anguished the most.

She was afraid to die – this was her anguish. Her agony had come at the end of a long and difficult struggle with cancer, the most difficult part of which, she had told me, was the mental depression, sadness and discouragement she had experienced as she became progressively weaker. But underlying all these difficulties, she confided, was her fear of dying. That she was coming to the end of her illness was clear to me and to her. Death for her, we both knew, was imminent.

Now, in her agony, her struggle was acute. Filled with self-reproach and inner torture, her distress was excruciating. Her whole body was restless, feverish, and agitated. Nothing helped her. Fear gripped her.

"Pray for me," she said, "I'm afraid … I'm so afraid to die."

I stood beside her holding her hand and prayed aloud, "Father, in the name of Jesus, we come to you and ask that you dispel from Lucy all that is not of you. Remove all fear and anxiety from her and fill her with your love and your grace. Mary, our Mother, be with her now and protect her from evil. St. Joseph, patron of the dying, intercede for her. Father, we ask, too, that all the effects of the Sacrament of the Sick received earlier today be operative in Lucy now as then. Amen."

As I made the sign of the cross with oil on her forehead, something happened to me. Suddenly I felt so repelled at even the thought of being with, to say nothing of praying with, Lucy, that everything in me wanted to run – wanted to run as far away as possible. Although I forced myself to hold her hand and to wash her face, everything about Lucy's dying disgusted me. Her breathing was labored and unbearably loud; and no matter how I positioned myself in the room, I felt her breathing directly into my face. It seemed as if I, too, had to take on death. I smelled it, I tasted it; her fear-filled anxious eyes, her clammy skin, her parched tongue – all these became part of me. I felt myself sink into death. I became death. I felt I died.

After some time, as though I had come through to the other side of death, I began to pray the name of Jesus to the rhythm of Lucy's breathing. As she breathed in the Spirit of Jesus, I prayed, "Je … sus." As she breathed out, I prayed, "Je … sus." This was all I did. No more.

There followed a great calm, a sense of peace: peace within Lucy herself; peace in the room; peace within me.

I no longer felt like running.

I felt free to go or stay.

I chose to stay. Lucy's final words to me, "I can die now," confirmed what I saw with my eyes and felt with my heart – that the torment, the anxiety and the fear had gone. Her deathwatch lasted only three hours and she remained peaceful to her last breath.

What released Lucy to take her last breath, it seems to me, was simply being present to her in such a way as to allow her to share weakness without judgment or condemnation. This manner of helping another move through the dying process is also noted by Dr. Elizabeth Kubler-Ross. She says that, when we help patients express their feelings without judging them and when these feelings are heard by one who wants to hear them, then they can move quickly through the death process.[3]

Despite the brevity of her deathwatch, it is Lucy who, by letting me seemingly die with her, has taught me the most about death. First of all, just as I allowed her to share her fear and anguish, so too, she allowed me to share my own struggle to stay with her. Thus, together we could suffer through the darkness in each of us and together we could die in peace.

Secondly, even the abhorrence I felt has helped me to grow in compassion for those who might feel the same distaste as I do. Perhaps this feeling of repugnance is why so frequently no one goes near the dying person or why those who do are reluctant bystanders. I have come to understand that my caring extends not only to the dying but also to the timid who want to help but feel useless and out of place.

Thirdly, I wonder, if the dying person feels the same repulsiveness toward death in herself that I feel? If so, and I am inclined to think that she does, how could I run from the one who is experiencing her own repulsiveness? If I go, who will stay? Would it not be an act of love to stay with her through all that agony? Here, to stay means to pray. It is as simple as that.

Finally, is the evil one, I ask, so anxious to have me run that he tries to set up within me momentary false barriers hoping to intimidate me into running away and leaving the dying person all alone? But there is no need to run. Jesus is the victor. One heartfelt prayer made in the name of Jesus can send the evil one to his place. To ask Jesus to lift the fear, the anxiety, the pain, from the dying person as we keep vigil, is frequently enough to put an end to all that militates against rest and peace for her.

But sometimes we who watch, we who keep vigil, have to share that anguish. I anguished with Lucy until there was no more to anguish. Then, having been heard, she could die in peace.

My God, my God, why have you forsaken me?

Case Three
I Thirst (John 19:28).

Just as Jesus thirsted to have his physical needs attended to, so too Kate thirsted for bodily comforts. Kate had been in the hospital for two months suffering from an incurable blood dyscrasia which had become progressively worse. The day I was with her, she expressed one little wish: "I want to go home."

Within two days of my visit with Kate, the doctors had decided that there was nothing more they could do for her and permitted us to take her home with a prescription to relieve her pain. "Kate," I said, "I'm going to make the rounds of all your friends here and tell them that you are home. Is there anything else you'd like me to tell them?"

"Yes," she said, "tell them to pray for me *now*."

It was four o'clock Wednesday afternoon. The first person I met was Ann. "Ann," I said, "I need help, Kate's just come home from the hospital. She wants two things: she wants all of us to know she is home; she wants us to pray for her *now*. Please help me get that word to everyone here."

"What shall I say to them?" asked Ann.

"Ask each one if she'd like to pray for Kate and *how much*. Say that we'll report later what their prayer seems to be doing for her."

"She came home to die," mused Ann knowingly as she wheeled herself from person to person gently announcing the need to watch and pray for Kate.

In the evening Ann and I made the rounds again. Some had offered a half-hour of prayer, others as much as two hours. We told them that Kate had received the Sacrament of the Sick, that she was dying, and that she wanted them to continue to pray as much as they could. We agreed to return to them in the morning to give them details of Kate's condition.

We ended this round by returning to Kate. Ann said, "Everyone of us is praying for you and will continue to pray during the night as we wake up and again in the morning. Don't be afraid. It's good to have you home."

"Home, thank God," sighed Kate.

"Home in your own bed, in your own room with your own sisters," I reflected. She nodded and said, "The pain is getting worse again. Pray with me."

"Lord Jesus," I began, "in your mercy lift out of Kate's body the pain that is there. Bring about the palliative effects of the medicine she has received and thank you for letting her know your peace and rest that come as her bodily pain is relieved." I held her hand.

As I sat there with her and looked at her surroundings, I realized with what care the room had been prepared for her homecoming. Not only was the floor scrubbed and polished, the bed carefully made, but in addition all the little things she cherished were there. In full view on the table was the picture of her mother beside the Bible just as Kate had always kept it. Under the pillow was pinned the small crucifix she had worn for almost sixty years. Within reach was a well-thumbed loose-leaf notebook called, "My Favorite

Prayers." Then, as if to complete the scene, a friend, fingering her rosary, tiptoed in, squeezed Kate's hand, prayed slowly one "Hail Mary ..." and then quietly left the room.

To make her comfortable, I did what I could – I gently rubbed her back, washed her hands and face, moistened her lips. With a straw, I gave her a sip of water. As I did these things, I thought of speaking with her about dying but recalled that several months earlier she had told me how she enjoyed today and did not worry too much about tomorrow; she had obviously long ago faced the fact of her finiteness. I had sensed, even then, the feeling of inner and outer peace about her. Now, I realized, the pain is gone; she no longer wants to talk; it is enough simply to attend to her bodily needs, to hold her hand, to pray silently in my heart that the peace continue to the end and beyond it.

What I saw with Kate I am seeing with each sister – she seems to know when her time has come. When she feels ready to die, she wants only little human comforts like her favorite pillow, a little tea, the touch of a hand. Dr. Kubler-Ross notices the same thing. She cites the example of a twenty-three-year old man who was dying. He told Dr. Ross that during the night he had experienced himself as riding on a train and that he had begged the conductor to stop the train one-tenth of an inch short of its destination. Dr. Ross interprets the man's experience by saying that in his symbolic language the train ride represents his life and the conductor represents God. The man is begging God for a tiny extension of time. When Dr. Ross asks him how she can help him with the one-tenth of an inch, he asks her to convince his mother to go home and bake bread and make his favorite soup. The mother went home, made the bread and soup and brought it to her son. He ate a bite of the bread and a little soup. Shortly after that, he lost consciousness and died peacefully.[4]

Bread and soup are what this man wants; Kate's longing is to come home; and for her that means to be in the bed she had slept in for seventeen years and to have the familiar things she cherishes close by. But, more than anything else, it means the presence of her friends and their deathwatch prayer.

Twenty hours after she had come home from the hospital, Kate died peacefully.

I thirst.

Footnotes
Case One
1. For an explanation of what is meant by praying "... in the name of Jesus ..." see Dennis and Matthew Linn, S.J. *Healing Life's Hurts*, (N.Y.: Paulist Press, 1978), p. 122.

2. The oil I carry with me is oil blessed by a priest for use by the laity. The blessing for this nonsacramental oil is found under "Blessings of Things for Ordinary Use" in the old *Roman Ritual*, translated by Philip Weller (Milwaukee: Bruce, 1964), p. 573. Lay people may take the oil home and use it in healing prayer for each other.

Case Two
3. Elizabeth Kubler-Ross, M.D., *On Death and Dying*, The MacMillan Company, 1969.

Case Three
4. Elizabeth Kubler-Ross, M.D., *Coping with Death and Dying, Lessons from the Dying Patient*. 1973. Teaching Tape #2.

Chapter 7

Compassion and the Christian Nurse*

Gill McLean, B.S.N.
224 Mack St.
Kingston, Ontario K7L 1P7 Canada

Practitioner

After qualifying as a registered nurse from Adenbrooke's Hospital, Cambridge, England, Gill L. McLean worked first on an oncology unit and then on a general surgery, urology and dental unit. She later completed a Bachelor of Nursing degree at the Welsh National College of Medicine, then joined the staff of a hematology/medical unit. She is currently working as a bereavement counselor and a home maker.

Journey of Integration

As a Christian nurse, I struggle to be kind, compassionate, and gentle in the face of human suffering and my own brokenness. My thoughts and feelings often contradict what I know to be true as I strive to become a Christ-centered nurse. In the following case, I illustrate my emotional and spiritual journey as I faced my inability to grieve following the death of a patient.

In my struggle, I learned the truth of Pail's words to the Corinthians:

> Praise be to the God and Father of our Lord Jesus Christ, the Father of compassion and the God of all our comfort, who comforts us in all our troubles so that we can comfort those in any trouble with the comfort that we ourselves have received from God. For just as the sufferings of Christ flow over into our lives, so also through Christ our comfort overflows (2 Cor. 1:3-5).

Goal and Context

As a Christian nurse I am caught in a paradox. On one side I expect myself to be kind, compassionate and gentle, able to enter and share in the suffering of others. On the other side is the reality that I often struggle with turbulent emotions, callous attitudes, my own unhealed wounds and my human limitations in the face of another's suffering. Overwhelmed and incapable of feeling, my emotions remain frozen. This case study explores the nature of *true* compassion through an experience of being present to a patient's suffering and facing my own inability to feel and to grieve. The context of this illustration is a hospital oncology unit.

---

* This article is excerpted from "Compassion and the Christian Nurse." *Journal of Christian Healing*, 13:1:23-26.

Case Illustration
The Patient's Process

Geraint, 54, was diagnosed with acute myeloid leukemia in September 1987. He and his wife, Risa, had three daughters ages 23, 25 and 28. During Geraint's hospitalization, Risa was a devoted companion. Her time was spent either sitting at his bedside quietly reading or she would be walking Geraint around the hospital complex. Although petite, Risa was Geraint's encourager and helper.

Before his illness, Geraint had been employed as a foreman in a steel works. A tough but gentle man, he found prolonged illness difficult to accept. Separated from the normal world, the periods of hospitalization undermined his sense of control and personal freedom. He was frightened of the unknown: the treatments, the tests, and the outcome of his disease. Seeking consolation and strength to cope with these *unknowns*, Geraint relied heavily on the intimacy of his family relationships and his friendships at the hospital. Fellow patients were a particularly valuable source of information and support. They were able to explain how things would feel, and Geraint felt safe within the spirit of camaraderie on the unit.

Geraint responded well to chemotherapy. His remission was followed by consolidation treatment, and then a bone-marrow transplant was scheduled. Geraint appeared to be making good progress. However, in reality, he was frightened, and wanted simply to forget about his leukemia and live normally again.

Geraint was admitted to the hospital for the pre-transplant preparations (tests, bone-marrow harvest, and the insertion of a central intravenous line). Because he was physically well, he had time to watch and think. One afternoon during his stay I sat and chatted with Geraint.

It was perhaps the first and only time Geraint really talked to me. We spoke for several hours, and he described the impact illness had had on his life - how it had affected his family and friends. He described the things that had helped him to cope with the treatment and hospitalization, and the things that had frustrated and upset him.

As Geraint shared his thoughts and feelings, the conversation turned to religion. Geraint had been brought up as a Roman Catholic. However, as he progressed through school and college, he drifted away from his faith. Later, following his marriage, he stopped attending church altogether. Illness challenged Geraint to reconsider his faith. He began to question his belief in God, his values, and his way of life. He chose to rededicate himself to the Catholic Church because, he said, "Faith becomes real when I can associate with the mother figure of Mary."

During the months of illness, prayer had become important to Geraint. Prayer gave him strength and courage. Moreover, prayer enabled him to deal with his anxiety and the everyday concerns of illness: "If there's anything really worrying me, the only thing that helps is prayer." Nevertheless, he remained fearful of death, and his fear was rekindled by every death he witnessed on the unit. Recently, a young man called Graham had suffered a prolonged and painful death. This had a profound effect on Geraint, and he recounted his experience to me:

> I've never seen anyone so ill. I went in there one day and
> He could hardly breathe. He was just panting for air.

Unable to say anything to Graham's mother, who sat at his bedside, Geraint just went into the room, hugged her and walked out. "It was the least I could do," he told me. Unfortunately, Geraint now lived with this picture of Graham engraved in his mind.

In February, Geraint was admitted to the transplant unit for a bone-marrow rescue. After his discharge home, he returned to the hospital twice each week to receive a transfusion of blood and/or platelets. Two months elapsed. Geraint, having assumed that his own bone marrow would resume normal functioning soon after the transplant, was unprepared for his continuing dependence on the supportive transfusions. His concern and tension mounted. Then his childhood psoriasis flared up, and, toward the end of May, he was admitted to the dermatology unit for intensive skin therapy.

During his treatment, Geraint became subdued and depressed. He withdrew behind a wall of silence. He was discharged home; however, his convalescence was brief. Three weeks later he was readmitted to the ward with pneumocystis. Despite aggressive chemotherapy, his condition deteriorated rapidly. Geraint went into renal failure, and, after suffering respiratory arrest, lapsed into unconsciousness.

I was on night duty. The ward was quiet as I neared the end of the evening ritual of medications and lights out. Risa ran down the corridor toward me, her face drawn and white. I knew her message before she spoke. Geraint had had a second respiratory arrest. I called for the resuscitation bag, locked the medicine trolley and ran toward Geraint's cubicle.

Time evaporated as Geraint lay motionless and insensible and his skin turned dusky blue. Jean, the hematology resident, arrived, and together we entered a nightmare. After fighting to insert an airway, we fumbled to assemble the respiratory apparatus. The oxygen point was hidden and inaccessible behind the tangle of intravenous lines that hung above Geraint like strands of transparent spaghetti. There was no space in the tiny room. We pulled the heavy bed away from the wall, flung aside the pillows that had supported Geraint's swollen body and began the respiratory resuscitation procedure.

A few minutes later, Jean and I watched as the final blip faded from the cardiac monitor. Geraint lay still. There was nothing we could do. I felt numb. The whole situation was absurd, for although I had expected Geraint to die, his death had come as a stranger to me (Plantinga 1988). I went outside to break the news to Risa.

Risa wept as we walked toward the cubicle, my arm around her shoulders. I left her to say goodbye to the body that was no longer Geraint. I said nothing, for words seemed an unwelcome intrusion.

I went in search of Jean. She was standing in the ward sister's office, staring out of the window at the blackness of night. We hugged each other for solace, and Jean sobbed. I knew she felt angry, confused, and inadequate because of her inability to save the man who had reminded her so much of her father. Jean's tears of pain and grief were a stark contrast to my own emotional paralysis, my inner emptiness. I forced a few stony tears to salve my conscience.

I completed the formal hospital procedures that follow a patient's death as Risa phoned her family. Her words hung in the air as she repeated her short message:

"He's dead! Your father's dead! He died a few minutes ago."

I tried to imagine her thoughts. Was she remembering the months she had nursed Geraint through his treatment, now all for nothing? I tried to comprehend her grief, a mixture of anger, bitterness, and deep sorrow for the man who had died after an apparently "successful" bone-marrow transplant. I tried to understand her sadness for the loss of her husband, the man who never lived to see the green beans he had asked her to plant only two weeks before, the man who never lived to celebrate with his youngest daughter when she passed her final medical exams.

Time became meaningless. The daughters arrived, and one by one they paid their respects to their father. All the traces of medical treatment had been removed, and an orange blanket now covered his form. A vase of fading chrysanthemums stood on the windowsill, a small and inadequate gesture of humanity and consolation. Geraint's prized belongings - his beloved teddy bear, his string of rosary beads, his Bible and prayer book - lay atop his dressing gown in the gray property bag. They were now unnecessary artifacts.

The registrar arrived and asked if cryoprecipitate had been given. I nodded. I was shocked by his callous attitude, and yet I also was strangely aware that I felt equally cold and clinical.

An hour later Risa and I were finally alone. We sat together in silence at the nurses' station. Risa, mistaking my silence for sadness, smiled at me and said, "You can cry if you want to; I know how much you cared." I returned her smile and mumbled a few hollow words, but inside I felt awful. How could I disclose my real feelings? My life supposedly was characterized by the fruits of the Holy Spirit: compassion, kindness, humility, gentleness, and patience (Col. 3:12), and yet here in the midst of profound sorrow, I felt nothing but a cold insensitivity. I couldn't understand myself. Why couldn't I cry?

Process

For three days after Geraint's death, I struggled with my feelings. Unable to accept or even understand my coldness, I experienced a deep spiritual guilt (Lebun 1988). In church that Sunday, I was frightened - could fellow believers see through my veneer of respectable humanity? Prompted by my feelings of alienation, I pleaded with God to take away my cold, hard heart and replace it with a heart of compassion. I waited.

The prayers of intercession came. Someone asked God to comfort and support all those who were suffering. Another person praised God for his sovereignty and faithfulness, thanking him for his assurance of love in all circumstances. Then came the words of Rom. 8:38 (NIV),

> For I am convinced that neither death nor life, neither angels nor demons, neither the present nor the future, nor any powers, neither height nor depth, nor anything else in all creation will be able to separate us from the love of God that is in Christ Jesus our Lord.

Once again I was on the ward ... A sequence of pictures flashed through my mind - Geraint's face, the cardiac monitor, Jean hugging me in the office, and Risa smiling at me, quietly giving me permission to cry. My tears of release and healing fell. Finally, I was able to weep for the man I had known for those few brief moments. As I cried, I asked God to forgive me, and then I committed Geraint to his care. The words of scripture had given me what I needed. In order to grieve, I needed to be reminded of God's love for me even when my heart was overwhelmed and callous. In order to gain release from my anger, I needed to know that Geraint was never separated from the love of God.

Discussion

In retrospect, this experience showed me how difficult it really is for me to understand and empathize with another person's pain and grief. Floundering to find words that express love and concern, I also struggle to comprehend my own turbulent and battered emotions.

In personal loss and grief, an individual can gain comfort and solace from

Christ's crucifixion, the assurance that God understands and shares in *all* their suffering (Plantinga 1988). However, after experiencing my own inability to grieve, I would take the scenario further and say that it is Christ's compassion living within us that enables us to enter into and share in another's pain. It is Christ's supernatural love working in us that liberates us and develops our human emotions to their full potential, equipping us to mourn. For in our natural state, our hearts are at times hard and "deceitful above all things" (Jer. 17:9, NIV).

In our simple humanness, separate from God's Spirit, we are incapable of changing our own hearts, and, therefore, we need to surrender our inner selves to God. This surrender allows the transforming power of God's love to be released in our lives and to fulfill our potential. Indeed, David Seamands proposes that self-surrender is "the answer to life" (Seamands, 1987, p. 131).

As humans we struggle between our emotions and our wills. Indeed, our feelings may contradict what we know to be true and will to do, and we are in conflict within our selves. It is this conflict that leads to the suppression of our created humanity. Seamands offers the following insight to those struggling with this inner conflict:

> When I am in conflict, the best thing I can do is to take my feelings to God in ruthless honesty and tell Him what they really are (Seamands, 1987, p. 130).

The experience I have shared leads me to echo those words of advice. Unable to mourn, I had to confess my coldness and hard-heartedness. I had to offer my paralyzed emotions to God, asking him to free me. Only then was I able to receive the release and healing of grief. In an encounter with God, I realized a small measure of his compassion, and I emerged with a new and gentler heart.

References
Plantinga, C. (1988). "A love so fierce." *Journal of Christian Nursing*, 5:2 (1988).
Lebun, E. (1988). "Spiritual care: An element in nursing care planning," *Journal of Advanced Nursing*, 13: 314-20.
Seamands, D.A. (1987). *Putting Away Childish Things*. Wheaton, IL: Victor Books.

Chapter 8

Healing Rites and Rituals for Nursing Care in a Changed World

Catherine M. Meadows, R.N.
56 East Hoover Ave.
Phoenix, AZ 85004

Practitioner
　　Catherine M. Meadows, R.N., Consultant, was a Certified Emergency Room Nurse from 1993-1998, when illness forced her to discontinue her practice within the hospital environment. She has worked in staff positions as well as in management. She has practiced in every nursing environment from a one-bed hospital in rural Hawaii, corporate hospitals, and an inner city *level one* trauma center. She also has worked as a "House Supervisor" as part of her management responsibility and therefore had the privilege of supporting nurses from all areas of the hospital. Catherine is also a certified Gestalt therapist and Spiritual Director. She is currently studying at the Chaplaincy Institute for Arts and Interfaith Ministries with the goal of working in multi-cultural environments as an ordained chaplain.

Journey of Integration
　　Spirituality has been a passion of mine since high school. I am a Roman Catholic, yet in my early adult years when *searching*, I participated in a number of faith traditions. I was baptized in the Holy Spirit at an Assembly of God church. Later, realizing that it was time to return to my roots, I became part of the Catholic Charismatic movement in 1973. Since then I have been involved in Catholic charismatic prayer groups and regional gatherings. In 1987, through the Hawaii Benedictine Monastery, I felt called to Spiritual Direction and completed a course of study. Nursing is, for me, a call to ministry.
　　On a hot summer night, I was driving home after a 12-hour shift as an ER clinician. During my shift I had cared for many critically injured patients, including six who had died. As I was driving along reviewing the day, I realized that while I could remember the face of the first patient who had died, I could not remember his name or the story of how he arrived at the ER. I was appalled. I had been with him as he died and *I couldn't even remember his name*. As I thought about this, I became aware that the depression and anxiety I had been experiencing had a reason – I was not grounded in my time at work. I realized that I could survive, psychologically, morally and spiritually, *only* if I could create a ritual or rituals to protect myself. I needed a

structured way to immerse myself in God's love for me and for my patients; a way to acknowledge and appreciate all of what I and my colleagues had done, and, when patients died, a way that would allow me to let them go into God's arms. In addition to feeling overwhelmed with critical patients' physical needs, I was also painfully aware of the fact that we were not spiritually supporting our patients of different cultures and faith traditions. I pondered over issues of *burn out* of staff as well as our apparent inability to provide a supportive safe place for those of other religious traditions. This resulted in my passion for spreading the word about the need for rituals as well as education about the new patient population that we are caring for in today's world.

Context

The author worked in the third largest trauma center in California for six years. This trauma center cared for 250 patients a day - 65,000 patients a year. It was also the regional burn center. It dealt with the consequences of gang-related violence, treated the victims of serious car accidents, and saw children who had suffered unspeakable abuse at the hands of their parents. It also treated the more "normal" types of emergencies such as heart attacks, strokes, and so on. Because it was the "County Hospital," the poor, the medically indigent, and those with Medicaid insurance comprised a large part of the patient population. Portions of these patients were from different cultures and religious backgrounds.

Nursing Workday Issues in Acute Care Settings

The reality of our profession is that it is inherently stressful. Of course, it was just as stressful twenty years ago. It was stressful during the Vietnam War. It was stressful during World Wars I and II, etc. The high level of stress associated with nursing is not a new phenomenon, it is merely the case that the stressors have changed. As nurses, we need to begin by taking personal responsibility for the fact that we *choose* to work in a profession that is stressful.

Perhaps not coincidentally, the word "stress" falls right between "strength" and "stretch" in the dictionary. The tools we need to function as nurses in a stressful environment entail both strength and the ability to stretch. Faith, our belief in God, is the gift we have that provides us with the strength to do God's will. The ability to stretch is given us by the Holy Spirit and allows us to move beyond what we think we can do - to say or do things that we once would have considered impossible.

New Variables that Increase Stress

Contemporary nurses are experiencing issues that once were non-existent.

Because of corporate and public administration values, patient assignments are now done "by the hour." In other words staffing is done using the following formula: the number of nursing hours allowed is equal to the total number of patients (the "census") multiplied by the amount of nursing hours allowed, by some acuity measure, per patient. The acuity (level of care required) is supposed to be built into this formula by varying the number of nursing hours allowed per patient in different types of conditions. The situation regarding appropriate ratios of nursing care hours to patient need is so serious that Registered Nurses are having to work through the legislative system to ensure that the nursing hours allotted to each patient are adequate to provide safe patient care.[1] Nurses can no longer depend on health care institutions to be proponents of good patient care.

Exacerbating the tensions created by the system of "managed health care" (in the context of a violent society) is a new stressor: the growing heterogeneity of the patient population. The typical patient population has changed from one consisting primarily of Christian peoples with a relatively small minority of Jewish and Native American persons to a population that is very diverse in terms of both culture and faith. Beliefs and practices of many patients that are normative in their own culture may conflict with the beliefs and practices normative for their care givers.

Methods of Healing and Protection

Most nurses know to pray for their patients and their peers. We know how to say a quick "Hail Mary" when we are in over our heads. We know how to read scripture and apply it to our work. These practices are certainly important, but I believe that we must go further. In addition to our usual religious practices we need to know how to create intentional rites or rituals that are unique to our individual needs. In this manner, we can cloak ourselves in an awareness of God's presence, thereby enabling us to create an environment in which the patient is able to feel God's presence.

Goal

Here I intend to illustrate, for myself and my profession, vital ways to create sacred ground for myself and for my profession so that nurses can be the healers that God calls them to be. Some rites and rituals are examined which serve as vehicles of intentionality to increase nurses' physical, mental, emotional and spiritual ways of caring for themselves in the midst of intense clinical practice. Also addressed is the issue of caring for people of different cultures and religions.

Methodology/Theology

In my role as manager, I was a one-member SWAT team. When critically injured patients were brought into the Emergency Room, I would assist the staff in the initial assessment and treatment. Once the initial treatment had begun, I would go to be with the family. While I was extremely focused on the patients and their families, as soon as one crisis had ended, I would be swept into the next crisis. I came to notice a look of bewildered pain on the faces of the staff at the end of the day and I felt the same pain in my own heart. I realized that I had not recognized my own emotional and spiritual needs for protection, nor sought for a way to have closure with each patient and family. I always left a bit of my heart with each critical patient, and I was running out of heart.

I created a ritual for myself that embraced three needs:
- the need for feeling safe and grounded,
- the need to recognize each patient I cared for as a child of God, and
- the need for closure with each patient situation.

This ritual framework became a means of praying in some very intentional ways about and around my work activities. When I arrived at work in the morning, I began praying the minute I left my car in the parking area. As I walked towards the hospital, I would ask God to place angels at every entrance - to protect all who entered the hospital, to protect all who were within the building, and to protect the community around the hospital. Once inside the Emergency Department I prayed for all the patients and staff in the Emergency Room and for the rest of the staff and patients throughout the hospital. I would stand in front of the control board on which the names of all patients would be printed, and pray for all of them, since I often did not have the opportunity to be with the non-critical patients. One aspect of my job was to meet the needs of the families of critically injured or dying patients, and, as I checked out the family room, I would ask for the grace to bring the presence of God into each situation I encountered. This initial covering of the Emergency Room and hospital took very little time, but for me it created a place of holiness - holy ground if you will - within which I would best be able to bring God's presence.

I would pray specifically for each patient I encountered and for his or her loved ones. I spoke a few words to each trauma patient, trying to reassure them in their terror. I could do this at the same time I was starting an IV or helping to stabilize a patient's condition. My prayers for the patient were silent for the most part although I would many times say something such as "Come on God - we need your help with this one." Making *casual* prayers such as this was acceptable to staff, and I believed it helped to ground them even though many might not explicitly recognize the *holy* in each patient encounter. I never left the bedside of a critical or dying patient without a short prayer to God to take them in his arms. My anxiety and depression lessened - I was experiencing closure with each patient.

Illustrations

A Traffic Nightmare Leads to Teaching Approach about Rituals of Protection

I had the opportunity to mentor this prayer approach to staff as a result of their reaction to what is still considered by the National Transportation Board to be the largest multi-vehicle accident that has ever occurred. The accident happened during terrible weather conditions of thick central California fog and a raging dust storm. It involved 154 injured patients and 8 deaths. Subsequently staff members were clearly showing signs of post-traumatic stress: anxiety whenever it was foggy or dust storms were occurring, irritability, nightmares, and a decreased ability to handle multiple stressors, which is a way of life in emergency nursing. In order to assist the staff we brought in a "Critical Incident Debriefing Team." When asked how I handled stress I described in general terms how I created rituals to make sure I had closure with each patient. At an *off work* function I had a nursing staff member come to me and ask for help in creating a ritual. His role in the emergency department was a senior staff RN. He was perceived by his co-workers as a mentor, both clinically and professionally. (i.e., By his actions he would teach staff how to deal with abusive patients, making sure to discuss his actions with them after an incident). His understanding of God was from a very conservative Christian faith experience. Using his vocabulary we worked together and created a ritual where he felt safe and grounded, felt loved by God and felt able to pass on the patients he treated to God. He then began teaching other staff members how to create rituals suitable for their understanding of God and spiritual practices. This, given the legal and union climate in which I was employed, was far more appropriate than me, as manager, teaching staff helpful rituals involving God. The staff felt free to approach him, he talked about his faith experience in a low-key manner and was not judgmental. He would come to me for assistance and we always made sure it was *off grounds*. Although we did not do a formal study of the results of this training, the anecdotal evidence was that the staff who created rituals appeared to be more present to their patients, and less stressed in the work environment.

Cultural and Religious Diversity

As healthcare workers, I believe it is our job to provide patients of any belief system the physical, spiritual and cultural support they need to promote healing. Huge gaps in beliefs and practices make this challenging. The aspect of the problem easiest to address is staff ignorance of the practices and beliefs of other cultures. Education is always a fairly easy cure for ignorance. More difficult has been the task of balancing traditional beliefs with medicine as practiced in a large emergency room in the United States; balancing respect of others' belief systems while still providing the patient with what we believed to be the best care. This is a difficult juggling act and can be done well only when done with as much knowledge and intentionality as possible.

The issue that arose, as the patient population became increasingly culturally diverse, was how to be present to people of other cultures in a spiritual way while neither compromising our own beliefs nor imposing them on others. Those of us who believed in the healing power of the Holy Spirit faced this situation with additional questions. As a group of us prayed and talked about this we came to some conclusions. One, we realized that by covering ourselves in the protection of Jesus, that we were in no danger. Two, we believed that God would be present to patients - our responsibility was to create an environment where that Presence could be experienced by our patients. Three, we studied and developed an appreciation of other cultures' experience of religion, which opened up the opportunity to begin dialoguing with others, even if not of our own belief system. Finally, we realized that our role was not to evangelize in the Emergency Room setting. Our role was to provide support. By turning over to Jesus the issue of how to spiritually connect with others of different beliefs, we were able to be true to our spiritual selves while trusting that God would take care of the bigger questions.

The Hmong

In our city we had a sudden influx of Hmong. Hmong are a shamanistic tribal people from the highlands of Laos. A shaman is a ritual or religious specialist who is believed to be capable of communicating with spirit powers. Most Hmong practice Theravada Buddhism. Hmong health care beliefs and practices are significantly related to Brahmanistic and animistic beliefs. In caring for the Hmong we learned that their perception of illness was that it could be attributed to the loss of one of the thirty two spirits thought to inhabit the body.[2] It is the Shaman's role to call back the lost spirit and therefore heal the ill person. These people were suddenly thrust into a world of which they could make no sense. They came from simple grass huts into the chaos of a large city. Their healing rituals included *coining* (rubbing a coin all over a sick persons body and raising welts) placing a chicken on a sick person to peck out evil spirits and other traditional rites. It was easy to see how staff, so firmly rooted in their own cultural beliefs, would come to the conclusion that a child who had been *coined* or *pecked* had been abused. The staff both ignored other cultures' ways of living and communicated strong disapproval of the different cultures' healing rituals.

An incident that raised everyone's consciousness about the importance of knowing another's cultural practices and beliefs, as well as any myths they might have about North American medical practices, was demonstrated in the case of a 37 year-old Hmong woman with four children. She was a member of one of the first groups of Hmong that emigrated to North America. On presentation to the hospital, she was diagnosed with advanced breast cancer with metastases in her lungs and brain. There were two issues that we struggled over - her level of treatment and her *code status*.

Initially she refused any treatment for her breast cancer. In her case, treatment would not have saved her, but it probably would have averted the suffering incurred by the large and painful wounds appearing before she died. As we talked with her and her family (via a translator – a whole other issue), it was clear that she believed she had *lost spirits* and she would either die or get well. Because of the family's belief system and the family's inability, as they began their lives in the United States, to make the distinction between extraordinary means of treatment and comfort means of treatment, she remained a *Full Code* (i.e., do everything possible to keep her alive if she stopped breathing or her heart stopped). The staff was frustrated because she was admitted many times through the ER and they watched as she wasted away - in pain. The family considered pain medication a way of interfering with the spirits. Finally, the physician managing her care and the Shaman (with the help of a good translator) worked with the family. They used traditional healing rites and educated the hospital staff at the same time so that this woman finally received the palliative she needed.

Discussion

I have talked about stressors present in the practice of medicine, some of which are relatively new. As moral beings, we must try to provide the best care we can in this context. Moving into a more corporate environment and *bottom line* mentality has made it so that nurses have to do more with less. We must become educated about the business world and come together as a united group to fight for the safety of patients. I have also addressed the stressors of caring for patients that are from other cultures and faith traditions.

Additionally, when a nurse's day may entail having to swiftly move from patient to patient, where each patient is experiencing what, for them, is a life-ending or life-changing serious trauma, we must both protect our own hearts and souls and provide a context in which patients can experience God's presence. It is my belief that by quietly bringing our own spirituality into the practice of medicine, we continue: to feel God in our lives, to appreciate the value of each person as God's child, and to bring God's presence to those experiencing pain *without* imposing our belief systems on others. By creating and practicing our own private rituals, we are better able to move with God's grace through the earthly suffering we see.

Finally, Jesus taught us that we ought not judge others. In our increasingly heterogeneous society, we must learn to help those whose spiritual practices are unknown and unfamiliar to us. We have an ethical responsibility to learn about the patient cultures we are encountering, and to bring God's presence to each patient while respecting the nuances of each person's belief system.

The most important message I hope to give is the need for personal ritual and intentionality. We need to create rituals, praying for protection, for ourselves, and others we meet. We need to recognize those things in our environment that are soul draining and put the light of Jesus around our souls. We need to be intentional, every day, in the practice of our spirituality. We need to be humble enough to realize that our lives as professionals are now more global and that we need to respect others and their belief systems. We must trust that God will take care of the rest.

References
1. California Nursing Association Information Publication 11/2000.
2. 1997 Laos Family Community of Minnesota, Inc.

Organizational Development

Chapter 9

Healing An Organization: A Case Study

Bonita Lay-Oliver, B.S., M.A.
Box 943 Road Town
Tortola, British Virgin Islands

Practitioner

Bonita Lay, B.S. Physical Education, minor in Health, Spalding University, Louisville, KY, 1970. M.A. Health Education, Adelphi University, Garden City, NY, 1975. Post Graduate Work in Health Promotion at Johns Hopkins University Hospital. Alcohol and Substance Abuse & Employee Assistance Programs at Georgia Technical Institute; Health Care Services Marketing at Georgia State University and Alcohol & Substance Abuse at Ohio State University. Certifications in Myers-Briggs Type Indicator; Benchmarks (Center for Creative Leadership), Greensboro, NC and American Arbitration Association, Labor Arbitrator and Mediator. Spiritual Direction Education at the Spirit Life Center, Plainview, NY.

Journey of Integration

This is my story of experiences that ultimately led up to the case study. It is important to include them as they gave me opportunities to test methods and to move to the *next steps*.

After a seven-year stint of teaching in mainstream education, my journey of integrating healing prayer and spiritual healing with organizational development began after my own healing from a spirit of self-hate in January, 1978. After that healing I felt that I was to become a *corporate apostle*. This is a term that I coined to help define a Christian mandate: to evangelize and to witness Jesus Christ as healer at the work site. This evolving ministry has progressed over a period of 20 years. Professionally trained initially as a health educator, I have evolved into a human resource systems consultant. The processes I have integrated include health promotion, health and wellness, change and transition models, career management, organizational development, marketing and quality. With this case study, the spiritual and prayer intervention component was an overt addition.

In July, 1978 I was hired as the first corporate health educator for Blue Cross and Blue Shield in the U.S. Due to the unacceptability of prayer in a public setting and even though it was a personal value, I would not use scripture or prayer at the work site. At the time, empirical research was just start-

---

* First published in *The Journal of Christian Healing*, Volume 21, Number 1, Spring, 1999, pp. 3-14.

ing as health promotion and wellness at the work site was quite new. A health insurance company hired me to help demonstrate that healthy people are more productive people. Specific people who worked with me developed pivotal research.[1] This research and the models of health promotion were springboards for the health promotion models used today. At that time, the only way for a business organization to buy into *healthy employees* was through *bottom line* issues, comparisons of the cost of health insurance premiums and lifestyle diseases. Although there was no drawback to that, health promotion and wellness takes into consideration the *total* person. The total person is mind, body *and spirit*. The spiritual component was not evident. Measuring the outcomes were sketchy at best.

Adding Additional Disciplines: Marketing and Human Resources
During the late 70's and early 80's, health practitioners in mainstream medicine (doctors, nurses, therapists, dentists, health educators et. al) would not have thought to integrate organizational development or even to combine marketing with health care. Professionals *just hung out their shingle* and did business. In my experience at professional meetings, there would be discussions about marketing but it was felt that marketers were *hucksters*. It was not until marketing professionals earned health degrees and health professionals earned marketing degrees that attitudes began to change. More bridge building developed between the disciplines and we now have Health Services Marketing as an integral component of Health Care.

Raised Eyebrows
During my tenure at my next job, working as a Community Health Services Director for a hospital in Atlanta, I was asked to participate in the 1980 International Diabetes Conference held at the Center for Disease Control (CDC) in Atlanta. I was asked to make a presentation on "Marketing Health Care Services."

As I was waiting for my turn to present, a nurse speaking before me was explaining how she was able to get Native Americans to come to their diabetes clinics with the lure of bingo and other games of chance. I realized the nurse was encouraging another negative health behavior, gaming or gambling, to a population that is known to be predisposed to addiction. This captured my attention since I was acquainted with the 12 step program of AA.[2] The 12th step states: "Practice these principles in all our affairs." This was the point where I began to integrate 12 step work in *all business and work site projects*. Addictive behavior (unless treated) can also be demonstrated through leadership in an organization, fostering co-dependencies (Ann Wilson Shaef, 1988). If an executive uses the 12 step program, (s)he must change the unhealthy behavior or else (s)he would revert back to the destructive behavior. The subordinates (employees) would then demonstrate co-dependent behavior in order to fit in as part of the team. This helps *define* organizational climate and culture.

Encyclicals as Guidelines
Because of my Roman Catholic background, I studied social encyclicals of recent popes. I specifically investigated what was written about *work*. I believe that these encyclicals are inspired by the Holy Spirit and that they contain information to help develop a more informed conscience. One encyclical in particular caught my attention. It has much to do with my evolving Case Study.

Pope Leo XIII, in his encyclical *The Condition of the Working Classes*,[3] alluded to the term which is used in Organization Development called ESOP's (Employee Stock Option Plans). Basically, this is where employees take ownership of their work. Since the English translation of this encyclical in 1942, this idea took about 40 years to become a workplace reality. The pope's footnotes were all biblical in nature.

This slow but sure response to Leo's teaching gave me courage and confidence to press on. I would now attempt to trust and follow the prompting of the Holy Spirit. In my own compartmentalized life I did not feel that I had an integration of my work with my prayer life. I feel that my listening to the promptings of the Holy Spirit to work toward that integration was facilitated through education, through a *Life in the Spirit Seminar*, and through Spiritual Direction.

Careers in Transitions
In the early to mid 80's, the onslaught of downsizing caught fire. I knew what other *downsized* persons were experiencing because I had been *downsized* as a tenured teacher in the 70's. I had experienced grief, loss, despair, and even age discrimination. I believed that by helping others process their grief, loss and pain, I too, would heal. At this point I had an opportunity to make a career transition to become a human resources professional and I began working in the Outplacement Industry teaching *downsized* persons to make career transitions.

Work is more than just a *job*. It is intimate and can be very life fulfilling. Focusing on these aspects of work gave me an opportunity to bring a Gospel promise "I have come to bring you abundant life" (John 10:10) to the workplace. I tried to give individuals an opportunity to *take stock*. They would identify their strengths through assessment and apply those strengths where they would be able to grow.

I also observed that persons who persist in a workplace position, may have to forego their strengths. Employees do use their skills, but may not engage their interests (things individuals *like* to do). Work, then is more in line with their God given talents. By focusing on their strengths and not their weaknesses, individuals can focus on achievement. They learn to set goals which are personal in nature. When individuals achieve more, the organization also meets its goals. These organizational goals include time management, productivity, sales and influencing skills and people skills.

Additional Programs

I was able to develop a stress management workshop for the Third Order of Franciscans in which I used an assessment that identified 19 different thinking styles[4] and their relation to stress. With this workshop, I researched and included biblical passages to add the spiritual dimension.

In 1995, a team-building experience at the Spirit Life Center in Plainview, NY solidified my hypothesis that spiritual healing in organizations could become a viable reality in the worksite by integrating prayer and organizational development interventions. The Spirit Life Center was going through accelerated growth at the time and team building was necessary for the various ministries to work more effectively together. I usually need two days to process a group for team building. Because of time constraints, the Director of the Center gave me a day and a quarter. When the Director used an hour of that allotted time for prayer and praise, I was anxious that I would not have enough time to complete the team building process. I was surprised at how efficiently and smoothly the process proceeded with the large group of 60 people. The Director was pleased with the results.

Context

The context of this illustration is an organizational healing ministry. The client was referred by another corporate client of Bonita E. Lay &. Associates Ltd.

Goals

The therapeutic goals of this case illustration were:
- To enhance wholeness and quality of life at the work site.
- To promote the health of employees.
- To provide interventions and prescriptions for organizational culture changes.
- To raise the level of cooperation and improve relationships within the organization.
- To help identify *next steps* for continued improvement.

Theology

Pope John Paul II states in his encyclical *Laborem Exercens:*

"In its subjective dimension, work is always a personal action. It follows that the whole person, body and spirit, partakes of it, whether it be manual or intellectual labor. The Word of the Living God, the evangelical message of salvation, is also directed to the whole person, for we find that many of the contents of that message are concerned with human work. They are like special lights shining upon it. There is need for interior effort of the human spirit, guided by faith, hope and charity, to give through the aid of those contents, the labor of the concrete man the significance which it has in God's eyes. Through this significance, labor enters into the work of salvation.

The Church considers it a duty to make pronouncements on work and the moral order to which it pertains. At the same time, she sees a particular duty of her own to form a spirituality of work, such as may help all people get closer to God and by its means, partake in his saving plans for man and the world and deepen friendship with Christ in their lives" [5] (*Lab. Ex. #24*).

Theory

1. Feedback and questionnaires gave me the information that my ideas to help with people issues at the work site were being assimilated at least intellectually. However, it became apparent that there was still something significantly lacking. There was not any spirit - *élan vital* (enthusiasm). Morale was still impaired. The organizations I worked with gave employees benefits, wage increases, had forums to hear complaints, suggestions and the like, but something was missing.

Since the culture where this case study takes place is quite open to the Spiritual/Christian dimension, I decided to integrate scriptural passages and spiritual elements into the process of change to facilitate healing. I could speak to Christian employees about Moses, the Promised Land, their *murmuring motif* (Let's go back to Egypt, at least we know what we had) and the need to move forward through organizational workshops. I used language, values and beliefs that were known to them and helped make the transition to incorporate the needed change within the organization.

2. Father George Montague, in the chapter "The Spirit and the Creative Use of Chaos" from his book *Still Riding the Wind*,[6] gave examples of bringing order out of chaos: In the book of Ezekiel Chapters 36-37, Ezekiel sees God's spirit coming upon dry bones scattered on a desert plain and bringing them back to life and Isaiah in Chapters 40:7-8; 42:1; 44:3-4 sees both God's spirit and his words as agents of a new creation. I wanted to integrate the organizational development process, with scriptural stories and various forms of prayer, i.e. praying with Christian employees and blessing them with holy oil. In this way I was able to help promote order out of chaos at the

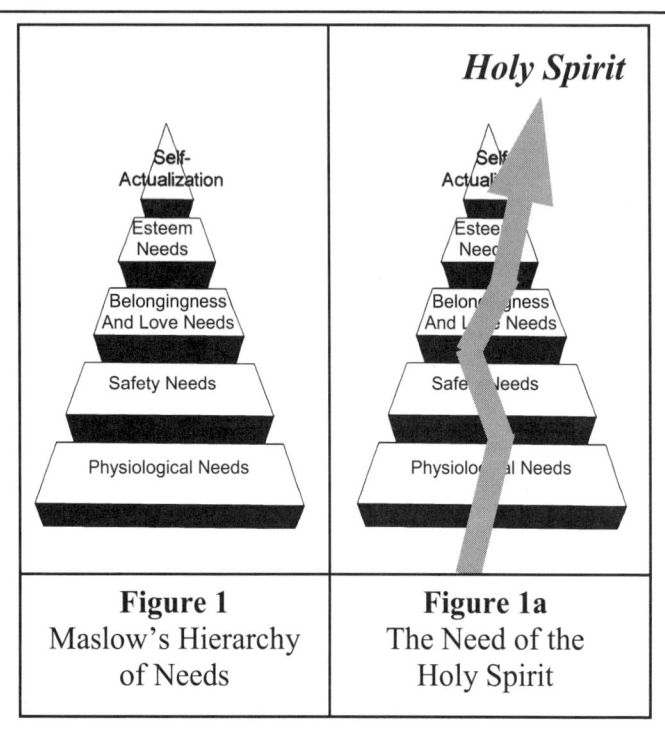

Self-Actualization Esteem Needs Belongingness And Love Needs Safety Needs Physiological Needs	*Holy Spirit* Self-Actualization Esteem Needs Belongingness And Love Needs Safety Needs Physiological Needs
Figure 1 Maslow's Hierarchy of Needs	**Figure 1a** The Need of the Holy Spirit

work site. These prayers included prayers of praise, prayers of thanksgiving and prayers of petition.

3. Abraham Maslow's "Hierarchy of Needs" (see Figure 1) is well accepted as a cornerstone in today's thinking on psychology. However, it is *humanistic*. What the model does not demonstrate is the influence of the Holy Spirit, the Power, the *Ruah* that actually transforms people and makes them whole. The Holy Spirit is not an intellectual power but a gentle, loving, yet dynamic impulse, similar to the function of the wind. The primary function of the Holy Spirit is not to give understanding, but to give movement, not to shed light, but to impart dynamism. Only the Holy Spirit knows our intimate reactions and thoughts not yet communicated with others. The concept of the Holy Spirit can give rise to some confusion, but it does bring a wealth of images. So, rather than clinging to an over intellectual and arid concept, we could take in its wealth. The bottom line is that the Holy Spirit is the creative breath of God[7] (see Figure 1a).

4. Chaos of any type can be transformed into promise if the Spirit of God is allowed to hover over it and when the Spirit has hovered sufficiently, the chaos responds in obedience to the Word, "Let there be Light."[6]

5. In this time in our history, more attention is given to the emotionally *poor*:

those experiencing divorce, relationship problems, alcoholism or other addictions. The integration of the spiritual dimension, namely the healing power of Jesus, offers Christian workers direction toward individual healing. As employees are personally healed, the organization itself can then become a healing environment, i.e. an atmosphere that lends itself to continue the healing process. Healing interventions for the organization would then include processes that would check on both the human resource development and develop the *quality* systems ensuring they are doing what they say they are doing.

Methodology
The following steps were used in this particular case.
- Spiritual preparation of the presenters by means of prayer, sacraments of Reconciliation and Holy Eucharist.
- Meeting with Senior Management to get an understanding of the issues and the problems at the work site.
- Meeting with Supervisors to include both Union and non-Union officials as a group so that they would understand the agenda.
- Identifying the spiritual position of the group as a whole.
- Posting an informal letter of agreement giving the limits of operation. All questionnaires and assessments produced would be displayed and intentions made plain. In order to reveal any information, employees need to feel psychologically safe. The supervisors, in accepting this, would sign the letter of agreement as symbolic gesture between participants coming from different stances.
- Demonstrating where and why the interventions happen.
- Explaining the change process.
- Initially carrying out one-on-one interviews; praying with individuals; identifying issues.
- Ensuring that all union and non-union supervisors receive the same copy of report that is sent to management.
- Identifying community resources for appropriate counseling.
- Deciding upon next steps.
- Determining specific training needs for staff and consulting with management.
- Carrying out follow-up training for employees dealing with supervisor behavior, task achievements and interpersonal skills progress, assessed by questionnaire.
- Evaluating data produced.

Case Illustration
Background and Initial Intervention

In 1995, I was asked to provide consulting and training services to a telecommunications company in Grenada, West Indies. This particular company is part of an organization that provides telecommunication services worldwide. I was concerned about the reception I would receive, given the anti-American sentiments after the 1983 *invasion* of the island. I felt strange, being a white American female approaching an organization that had all the usual organizational issues plus Marxism. I made it plain that I had only heard one side of the story about the invasion, that given by CNN and President Reagan, and was keen to hear their views. It was humbling for an American to learn that all people do not necessarily flourish under a democracy. My prayer life, including daily Mass was an essential component in facing these stresses. I completed my work and then returned home to the British Virgin Islands.

Providential Happenings

In October 1997, I received a phone call from the *company* asking me to provide consulting and possibly some training on the recommendation of the previous client in Grenada. This new client initially requested a "Customer Service" focused program. Their perceived problem was a total breakdown of relationships, trust and communication between management and employees. My assignment was to determine what the situation was by one-on-one interviews and then report back.

What Was Wrong

The result of my eventual investigation was that, even though the organization was functioning and not losing money, it was "bleeding and leaking" all over. The organization was one of the most complex that I had ever encountered. It interfaced directly with Customs and the Police (Government Agents), Shipping Agents (Private Enterprise) and the General Public, affected by local, regional and international laws of shipping which sometimes contradict one another. The demographics of the *company* were 98% male, comprising one General Manager, four Senior Managers and nine Supervisors (three of which were Union Stewards). The rest of the employee population was split union/non union. Influences of Democracy and Marxism were in coexistence.

The Assignment

In November 1997, I flew to Grenada. When I arrived, as my planned work schedule would not allow me to attend Mass, I arranged to receive Communion as part of my daily prayer. These were also moments for inter-

LEVEL I — Content: Work to be done

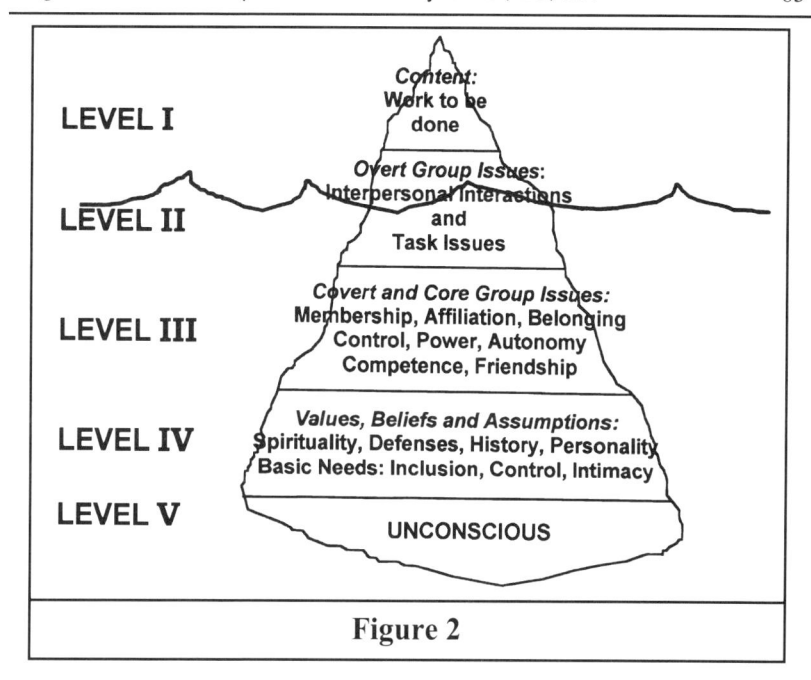

LEVEL II — Overt Group Issues: Interpersonal Interactions and Task Issues

LEVEL III — Covert and Core Group Issues: Membership, Affiliation, Belonging Control, Power, Autonomy Competence, Friendship

LEVEL IV — Values, Beliefs and Assumptions: Spirituality, Defenses, History, Personality Basic Needs: Inclusion, Control, Intimacy

LEVEL V — UNCONSCIOUS

Figure 2

cessory prayer.

The Beginning: Initial Interventions

On Monday morning, I met the general manager. He told me that he had a reputation for being, and was, authoritative and dictatorial. He punctuated this by blowing cigarette smoke in my general direction. I replied, tongue-in-cheek, that he could be sent to a charm school for bullies. I think he liked this direct approach.

I next met with the union stewards and supervisors. I initially wrote an agreement on a flip chart that all employees would be psychologically safe to talk to me. Whatever was said would be in confidence. They would also receive the same report that I would send to management. This was an effort to keep all of us honest especially in this non trusting environment.

As I went about interviewing the employees, I noticed that many of the men wore crucifixes. I felt that I was face to face with their spirituality, their values and their beliefs. Now, whether it was decorative or not, I decided to ask them if I could pray with them. They agreed. I was moving into a much deeper level than is customarily accessed by an organizational consultant - Level IV of Figure 2. Little did I know at that time how my knowledge and training within the Healing Ministry was going to be called upon. After prayer and anointing with blessed oil, these employees felt safe enough to share with me their life traumas. These included: incest, physical and emotional abuse, addictions, one employee with possible Dissociate Identity Disorder (DID), and a general *not at peace* demeanor. All of these issues surfaced as we tackled the typical human resource questions such as job satisfaction, what they did or did not like about their jobs etc.

I was also gathering more detailed information and continuing to build rapport. These efforts included:
- Identifying critical success factors, as seen by the client at the time.
- Understanding and appreciating the world the client comes from and the reality and perceptions within which it operates.
- Further assessing and clarifying the real issues as they continue to surface, seeking to dramatize natural tensions and discrepancies as appropriate.
- Acknowledging differences and understanding the implications of those differences.
- Helping clients reflect on their motivations for change.
- Being aware of how my own biases can influence the process (!)
- Identifying informal and formal power in the client organization in order to gain further commitment and mobilize people in a common direction.
- Ensuring that the process would not leave the organization in worse shape than when I came.
- Having a high tolerance for the unknown.
- Energizing others and oneself.
- Being skilled in handling diversity and diverse situations.
- Developing relationships at all levels that are grounded in trust and credibility.
- Seeking commitment and participation from all those affected within the organization.
- Dealing effectively with resistance as it surfaces.
- Mapping out a plan for managing the process.
- Recognizing the skill level required to solve a long-standing problem or recurring/ongoing conflict.
- Maintaining a tolerance for working through the process, especially when things grow complex or emotionally charged.
- Using my spiritual foundation and inner power sources for the benefit of the client and their realm of influence.

The process continues to determine the appropriate skills needed for collecting data; to document the current condition; to analyze and interpret relevant data; to provide useful and focused feedback; to provide Action/Intervention planning and the actual Intervention, Evaluation, Adoption and Separation.

By Tuesday afternoon, I was alarmingly concerned. There were limited opportunities for individual counseling on the island and most were government sponsored. Confidentiality was an issue. One female employee, who I believed to be a DID (Dissociative Identity Disorder), showed severe depression with suicidal tendencies. The Management complained that they could not figure out who this female employee was as she demonstrated quite a few personalities and was incorrigible. I also did not find compassion or empathy for emotional disorders from the general manager.

At the end of the day, I walked from the work site to my hotel to help clear my mind. Upon arrival at the hotel, I met a gentleman who asked me what I was doing in Grenada, identifying himself as a senior executive in government. I told him I was working with *the company*. He then related to me that he and the general manager had grown up together and when the general manager was a lad, he had witnessed his father murder his mother. The information, if true, helped me understand the general manager's behavior. I confirmed it's veracity through a friend and the personnel officer.

On Thursday, the general manager called a staff meeting and wanted me to address the employees. It was not part of our agreement, but I decided to take advantage of the opportunity. The union president opened his Bible and started with a scripture reading. When it was my turn to talk, I asked the union president if I could use his Bible and read John 5:1-8 (The healing of the man at the pool of Bethesda). I asked the group if they wanted to get well and they said, "Yes." I then prayed quietly in tongues because I did not want my ego or logic to get in the way of what God wanted to accomplish. Praying in tongues is Scriptural. It was a mechanism to allow the Holy Spirit to work through me. As I went on with my presentation, I realized that my own father had worked for and retired from a very similar organization. This was a common bond I had with this company.

Following that meeting, the union members asked to see me separately. They asked that we pray. These men were also spirit-filled. We said a binding prayer against all spiritual attacks. This is a prayer that asks to hold together any negative or sinful influences and petition the Lord to remove them. We also prayed for discernment of spirits and for deliverance from spirits of chaos, mistrust, disunity and fear and then finally a bonding prayer. This is a prayer that asks the Holy Spirit to fill us with the spirit of peace, trust and unity in the name of Jesus. They then felt comfortable working with me. Any person can pray these prayers. These are not difficult concepts to understand since we deal with negative and positive spiritual factors all the time. Persons outside the experience of Catholic charismatic renewal would benefit from a *Life in the Spirit Seminar*.[9] This seminar gives the understanding, the authority and power to do these interventions.

The general manager did not know that I knew about his history. I made mention to him that the employees were bringing their trauma and dysfunction to the workplace and that they needed help. Blowing smoke again, he said that was unfortunate, however he would like me to come back.

I was able to connect the female employee with a priest for some counseling and for referral to appropriate psychotherapy. I called a priest because I had no other resources to suggest since it was my first time on the island. The employees did not trust the government-sponsored counseling service or the government mental health providers. The priest was able to refer the employees to different ministers or health care providers.

Mid Course Interventions

Early in the summer of 1998, I went back to Grenada. I told the personnel officer that I would like my work at *the company* to be a case study for the Association of Christian Therapists entitled "Healing an Organization." This visit was for in-depth staff development and supervisory training; additional counseling; and finding and meeting community resources. My original view that the organization was convoluted, complex and environmentally dangerous was reinforced. The company's physical compound was dangerous. There was consistent movement of hazardous materials on the premises since the company was located at a shipping port. It was quite dusty and there were problems with pigeons and rats. The men often settled their disagreements with physical violence. Each of the agencies within this compound had different rules and regulations, which made an unfair and uneven *ball park*. However, the supervisors were committed Christians and they were comfortable with allowing me to lapse into spiritual dialogues within the normal human resource rhetoric. I delved into their value and belief systems by discussing the possibility of changing their principles and relating them to Scripture. I would ask the participants for their insight and feedback. In a way, with my Christian rhetoric I could speak their *mother tongue*. The only justification for using this approach was that I had their permission to do so. We prayed a binding prayer and bonding prayer each time we stopped for breaks. We looked at diversity in the group and examined how it added to creative solution development. The whole of one session was spent setting the stage and praying together. (I remembered my experience at the Spirit Life Center where an hour was spent in praise and prayer before getting down to the work of team training.) As we prayed I noticed that my consultant's foot was tapping. I certainly have found that it is good to *give more time than is necessary to the Lord*.

Diversity

During the coursework for this company, one of the topics discussed was Stress Management. I used a module that I had previously developed for the

Third Order Franciscans for training in dealing with stress, with its inventory of thinking styles and passages from Scripture. From the discussions, they were able to grasp the concepts because they were able to understand the spiritual components.

We also did an exercise to identify their strengths. A particular weakness of the members of this group was to focus on negative aspects and not identify their true talents and strengths. An exercise on how to identify these strengths consisted in naming preferences, values, motivators and their favored work culture. Group members each had to identify six work accomplishments, things they were proud of, whether the organization had given them recognition for these or not. The bottom line was that they had to feel good about themselves. They had to demonstrate what skills they used, what were the results, and the benefits to the organization. Next they were asked to list what they felt they did well and what they liked to do.

Most people, doing this exercise, have a great deal of false humility. They feel that it is egotistic to talk about themselves with pride. However, in order to benefit organizations, employees must be able to communicate their strengths and how they can help the organization obtain their goals. The employees of this company resembled flowers blooming as they participated in this process. They named their gifts and were learning to give.

As the week went on, a potential union/management issue developed within *the company*. It had to do with whether or not an employee did or did not do what the contract stated he should do. It initially appeared like a grievance. I decided it would be an *on the spot* learning activity for me and took up the request for help. Before the class started, feelings were quite heated. I knew that if we had a chance to pray we could move towards defusing the situation. One of the participants was astute enough to remind us of this. We stopped, and we prayed. We asked for guidance, for wisdom, for clarity of thought, for discernment and for peace. The *rewards* of prayer give a hostile situation calm and peace. We felt Jesus' presence among us. As the facilitator, I brought out the direct and confrontational questions that could have been detrimental to the group's progress. I asked if the employee breached the agreement. One of the non-union supervisors thought I was trying to goad the situation. He wanted to talk to me outside the classroom. I said, "No," since we had developed an element of trust. We would resolve it there. The situation was openly discussed. The problem was identified and resolved without a union/management grievance.

Another topic in supervisory training was "Dealing with Trouble, Addiction and Sexual Harassment." Most management consultants are trained *not* to reveal their personal lives. Through my participation in the Association of Christian Therapists, I had learned the significance of the wounded healer. I used my personal example of how to deal with an alcoholic spouse to demonstrate that they needed to know community resources, including religious resources, to deal with such issues and refer their workers to such resources. Resources for healing, conversion and transformation would be needed.

At a "side bar", a course participant asked me how I had handled my experience. I started to talk about *Al-Anon* and the ACOK (Adult Child of the King)[10] program, a 12 step Catholic Charismatic program. There *is* hope to heal. I prayed with the person and a priest was again asked to help.

Since the union president was Pentecostal, I gave him Fr. George Montage's Book *Still Riding the Wind*. I pointed out the chapter on chaos. I marveled at the evangelical and spiritual power this group had to be channeled for the building up of individuals. Individuals make up the organization. The system within the organization needed assistance.

Outcomes

This disparate group agreed to form a supervisors' forum. They established rules on how they were going to operate. They opted to make decisions on a consensus basis. They would start and end all sessions with prayer. They promised to pray for and with each other. They realized they would not see eye to eye at all times, but they understood that their different talents and different strengths would give the organization a more dynamic and cohesive image to both employees and management. In order to monitor this newly formed behavior, questionnaires were sent to *the Company* for a *post operative check up* and evaluation before a subsequent visit.

Long Term Outcomes

The long-term result for the organization was a customer service focus with employees each appreciating each others' contributions and diversities. They manage their careers better by keeping a journal of their accomplishments as it relates to their job descriptions. They can have a greater control of their lives through goal setting. Individually, they were able to identify and recognize their gifts, and applied them in different capacities. They were in the process of identifying resources in the church community to help with spiritual direction and counseling for the employees. It was my hope that the participants would be able to continue with a *wellness* development process. Jesus *always* gives us a spiritual healing. He is asking for a deeper commitment and communion with him.

Discussion

The usual resource consultant's targeted area is directed toward level III on the chart in Figure 2. In this project the area targeted was spirituality on Level IV.

Change is ongoing. It can be uncertain. Dealing with issues never dealt with before and especially not having research to back it up can be construed as circumspect. Prior to this assignment, I had an opportunity to report on how a volcanic activity and individual stress were measured (Stress Management for employees living in Monsterrat with an active volcano and using Change Management and Stress Management Modules for Business Changes due to the devastation from Hurricane Marilyn). I realized that there was a need for dealing with ongoing physical uncertainty. I was able to synthesize a *one of a kind* treatment plan for these employees. These people were left with *nothing*. This led to the introduction and invocation of the Holy Spirit at this work site and unleashed new life. Out of the chaos came new life.

The employees were given additional assignments to help them in their newly formed behaviors using a SWOT analysis (Strength, Weakness, Opportunity and Threat). This is a generic management tool. It was also recommended that they keep a journal for review of progress. Interestingly enough, management within the organization felt that they did not need training, intervention or coaching. However, if the supervisors maintain their progress, the managerial staff will need their own training and interventions.

The supervisors and employees were taught skills of how to communicate and get what they needed and to do what they could within the context of their own job responsibilities. Community resources were identified for the employees to use.

Applicability

As in the medical profession, human resource and management consultants can use prayer as part of their intervention for healing and transforming an organization. Every organization has its culture and that culture may need transformation from years of systematic behavior. Change is imminent and this process was not used as a "management theory *de jour*."

This case study reflects a paradigm shift for the work site. It is a faith dimension. I did not move into any esoteric area, but only into prayer. Everything spiritually used was used in the tradition of the Catholic Church supported by Scripture. It is a test experience and any further study is encouraged.

As in Philippians Ch. 2:1-4, 14-18, we are Jesus' servants, *and* without competition. We are Jesus' shining examples of what can exist at the work site. I initially would have found this difficult to do in the United States but, if anything, it gave me hope and courage and to listen to Pope John Paul II: "Do Not Be Afraid!"

Reference Notes
1. Cioffi, J. (1980). *The Effect of Health Status Feedback on Health Beliefs:*

An Inquiry into the Prebehavioral Outcomes of a Health Hazard Appraisal. Doctoral Dissertation, Georgia State University.
2. *Twelve Steps and Twelve Traditions.* New York: Alcoholics Anonymous World Services, 1953.
3. Leo XIII. (1942). *Rerum Novarum (The Condition of the Working Class.)* as translated by The Daughters of St. Paul.
4. Human Synergistics International. (1994). *Stress Processing Report.* Plymouth, MI.
5. John Paul II. (1981). *Laborem Exercens.* Boston, MA: Pauline Books and Media.
6. Montague, G. (1994). *Still Riding the Wind: Learning the Ways of the Spirit.* (revised edition) Mineola, NY: Resurrection Press, Ltd.
7. Montague, G. ibid.
8. John Paul II. (1996) *The Spirit Giver of Life and Love: A Catechesis on the Creed.* Boston, MA: Pauline Books and Media.
9. Human Synergistics International, ibid.
10. ACOK (Adult Child of the King). Spirit Life Center, 300 Washington Ave., Plainview, NY 11803.

Additional References

Covey, S.R. (1994). *First Things First.* New York: Simon &. Schuster.

Covey, S.R. (1989). *Habits of Highly Effective People.* New York: Simon &. Schuster.

Dougherty, R.M. (1995). *Group Spiritual Direction.* New York: Paulist Press.

Libert, H. (1990). *Miracle in the Marketplace.* Mineola, NY: Resurrection Press.

Linn, D., Linn, M. and Fabricant, S. (1984). *Praying with Another for Healing.* New York: Paulist Press.

Shaef, A.W. and Fassel, D. (1988). *The Addictive Organization.* San Francisco: Harper Collins.

Sofield, L., Juliano, C., Hammett, R. (1990). *Design for Wholeness.* Notre Dame, IN: Ave Maria Press.

Sullivan, J.E. (1994). *The Relentless Hunger.* New York: Paulist Press.

Tournier, P. (1957). *The Meaning of Persons.* New York: Harper & Row.

Psychotherapy Practice

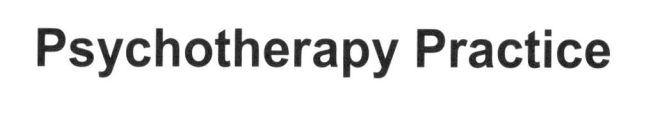

Chapter 10

Relational Presence and the Eternal Perspective

Karen Kozica Cichon, Ph.D.
1519 W Jackson Blvd.
Chicago, IL 60607

Practitioner

Karen Kozica Cichon received her Ph.D. in Clinical/Developmental Psychology and MA in Developmental Psychology from the University of Illinois at Chicago. Her BA, in Sociology and Psychology, was from Northern Illinois University. She interned at Northwestern University Medical School Outpatient Psychiatry Clinic and Children's Memorial Hospital, Chicago. She is presently studying at Catholic Theological Union.

Karen's professional development has continued mainly in the theoretical areas of Kohut's (1976) Self Psychology, Bowen's (1978) Family Systems, Erickson's (1994) Life Stages, and the Relational Psychology of the Stone Center. Besides an ongoing private practice, her professional experience has included providing consultation, training, and supervision at various Christian counseling agencies and teaching in Loyola University's Masters in Pastoral Counseling program.

Journey to Faith in Practice

It was in the middle of completing my complex and unwieldy doctoral dissertation, a seemingly endless struggle, that I experienced my adult conversion, reshaping truth as I had known it. The fundamental assumptions of the humanistic theories I was using in my study of Kohlberg's stages of moral judgment were awash in the tide of my new Christian worldview, rendering me functionally paralyzed. I eventually recovered, but I was never the same.

The change in my understanding of the nature of reality begged for a concomitant change in what I was doing in my psychotherapy practice. The books on healing and inner healing were not enough. I hungered for others who were on the quest and was finally directed to the Association of Christian Therapists (ACT) in 1981.

ACT has provided the fertile field necessary for the revelation of many forms of healing based on both sound spiritual and psychological principles. These have emerged not just through prayer, study, and discussion but through the process of ACT members experiencing and sharing personal healing journeys as well. Since, in psychotherapy, it is so true that *the medium is the message*, the personal transformation of the therapist has to be the start of any integration of faith into the therapy setting.

Part of the journey has included movement from those initial high expectations of miraculous healings, based on knowing the words to speak to a God we had experienced, through the disappointment of seeing much suffering go unabated. This has challenged my understanding and grown my faith. Today, I continue to move into a more contemplative mode of being with my patients and God and seeking his direction, including if, when, and how to pray.

Theology

For me, the essential question in psychotherapy, as in life, is: what is the true nature of reality? What makes the therapy I practice essentially Christian is a belief in what I call the *eternal perspective*; that the truest level of reality is spiritual, as well as natural, and that all we suffer here must be seen through that eternal perspective in order for us to apprehend the meaning of our lives and to know how to live. Hence, I see therapy as a spiritual journey, where we live out the Incarnation in our attempts to see God's truth in the struggles of our lives.

It is in *how* we see that we are moved and where change is possible. It is how we perceive ourselves in relation to the world that limits or empowers us. Enlarging our vision to include the Kingdom of God allows us to begin to comprehend our true identity and purpose in life. Without this grounding, human suffering is an incomprehensible evil, unattached to any greater meaning. The goal of Christian psychotherapy, then, is to "make straight the way of the Lord;" to remove the false realities which constrict peoples' ability to cooperate with God's grace and direction in their lives. It is about ministering the love of God to the dark places of the soul to set the captives free.

Some of the most fundamental beliefs that undergird my work, aside from, of course, the main tenets of orthodox Christianity, are that every person is created in the image of God in order to be in relationship with God in both his transcendent and his imminent manifestations. In God, we are one with one another, interdependent and interconnected, across time and space. To live in this awareness, which is to live in the Spirit, transforms our lives. We are impelled to grow in wholeness because it is clear that we were made to love; and we are empowered to reach into the eternal and become part of the divine plan of redeeming the world.

Clearly, I see conversion as the greatest healing because it is the revelation of the truth that sets us free, no matter what suffering we still have to bear. What happens in the therapy setting can range from healing on the level of simple relief of pain or meeting a human need, to freeing a family from generations of oppression. All of it, however, is done that we may be "perfect as our heavenly Father is perfect," one in justice, love, and mercy.

A Cautionary Note

Despite my heavily ministerial outlook, the most spiritual aspects of my work are not necessarily overt. After discerning whether there is a good fit between us, I enter into relationship with the person, both as a patient or client, and as a fellow traveler on life's journey, whose travels I am being asked to facilitate. In most cases, the person has come seeking help of a specifically Christian nature, greatly simplifying communication between us because of similar worldviews and language. The meanings and understandings behind the words, however, cannot always be assumed to be the same. Many people are seeking solutions to interpersonal problems through a deeper integration of God's ways into their lives, or, basically, Christian counseling. Many others, however, are more wounded, carrying the distortions from their earliest years into their relationships with God and Church and requiring deeper psychotherapeutic interventions. Until the therapist has a clear grasp both of the nature of those distortions and of the person's personal theology and spirituality, I believe it most professionally responsible to be very cautious about using overt religious interventions. The primary purpose of the therapeutic relationship is for psychological help, and clarity about the nature of the relationship, its boundaries, and transference issues, take ethical and therapeutic precedence over the personal expectations and desires of either the person seeking help or the therapist. For this reason, and in order to expand the capacity of the person in their own prayer life and in their ability to engage the resources of their faith community, I do not typically pray with my clients. If they are able, we talk about what issues need prayer and how to pray for them and who might pray with or for them.

That said, however, I must also admit to a larger view of prayer as being in active relationship with God and, in that sense, I strive to make prayer the constant ground of every session. The leading of the Holy Spirit and the centrality of the Lord in the work itself is acknowledged as a given. Scripture is the primary resource for discerning how to move through life's challenges, its imagery as well as its words providing new ways of responding and understanding.

Integration with Psychological Theory

This integrated approach offers a contemplative, faith-based understanding of depth psychotherapy which emphasizes being an appropriate, empathically-attuned presence to the other, mirroring the love of God for the person, and allowing oneself to be merged with God as a mediator of God's wisdom and power. This approach employs concepts from both Self Psychology and Relational Psychology to explain how the use of prayer, Scripture, and other Christian traditions and concepts, such as the Body of Christ and the Communion of Saints, can serve to call a person suffering from a depleted or disordered self into an experience of personal wholeness, with a life of meaning and purpose.

In the terms of Self Psychology, I believe that God gives himself to us as the Ultimate and Perfect Selfobject. His faithful, loving gaze mirrors us into eternal being as unique selves. His accessibility to us allows us to merge with his power in an idealization which will never disappoint. He offered us his Son as a brother, one who is like us and whom we are to become like. In Christian therapy, we mediate and facilitate that relationship for the person seeking healing. Just as we *loan our egos* to those attempting to build their own, so our faith serves as the bridge in healing the wounded spirit and bringing the personality to new life.

Empathic attunement is key to maintaining the therapeutic relationship and restoring connection in the therapeutic relationship when it is broken. It is through this movement of repeated attempts to come to accurately know, acknowledge, and respect the emerging person and their needs and desires that safety and trust are built and a healing relationship is made possible. Likewise, the therapeutic revelation of the trustworthiness of God, through his promises in Scripture and his actions in contemporary life, is a repeated process in the growth of faith and trust that is essential to a secure life. To establish the bond of shared experience with Jesus' life on earth and that of all the saints to the present time further grounds the person as one who belongs to something much bigger than the self. It is here that existence becomes significant and purposeful and that the deepest of human needs are met.

Case Illustration
Goal
To increase self-cohesion, self-acceptance, and capacity for trust and relationship in a chronically depressed and personality-disordered young woman.

Methodology
While the therapeutic process is similar in all my work, this case was chosen partially because it exemplifies how I use prayer in those instances where it has become a regular part of the therapy. The following description then, while generalizable, is written as specific to this case.
1) *Reconnection*: From the first glimpse in the waiting room, there is an ongoing assessment of the client's state of being and readiness to interact, including mood, issues, and themes, particularly as they relate to the therapeu-

tic relationship itself. The initial period of the session is spent negotiating through these in order to clear the path to connection so that inner work may begin.

2) *Empathic attunement*: By responding to the client's truest feeling state, I attempt to achieve and maintain connectedness with her. Because she both needs and fears closeness, I must prove myself trustworthy each session by being as relationally present as possible while allowing adequate space - getting a respectful distance right to allow for intimacy to occur.

3) *Deep listening*: Once the bond holds, there is a time of exploration of core issues, needs, and fears, during which I make gentle, tentative clarifications, assessments, and interpretations, relating what has come forward to other life and faith contexts - all leading to how we are to pray.

4) *Scriptural grounding*: We refer frequently to Scripture as the standard of truth; a piece that has become important in relieving the guilt of the overburdened self and giving permission for new behavior which often feels too good (dangerous) and creates anxiety over the potential for shame. Scripture is also an important source of healing images.

5) *Healing prayer*: Usually during the last 10-15 minutes of the session, we open up the wounded area to the healing touch of Jesus and pray accordingly.

6) *Faith imagery*: Most often, the prayer brings healing images, sometimes to the client and, almost always to myself, which express the current issue and the relationship of the self to God and others. These may then be worked with toward resolution.

7) *Separation*: Ending the session without disconnection requires multiple forms of reassurances communicating the permanence of the bond, such as recognition of and interest in life events that will be occurring in the client's life before the next meeting.

Client's History

Rachel is a 41 year-old woman who has been in therapy with me for chronic depression, self disorder, and related relationship issues, for much of her adult life. When she first came for help, she was defensive, angry, somewhat dissociative, and full of self-loathing. She could not take joy in any of her accomplishments and could not maintain mutually satisfying relationships. She was in constant ambivalence about being in the session and denied her own initiative in life.

Rachel was the eighth child in a family of twelve, with a depressed, withdrawn mother and a dominating, self-centered father. She has never been married and lives alone with multiple pets. She has worked steadily as a medical social worker and has recently completed her second graduate degree. Aside from her entrenched depression, she was diagnosed with lupus several years ago and has a variety of associated medical problems.

Rachel's childhood was marked by a tumultuous family life lacking in any stabilizing parental control or nurturance. Siblings were not safe from one another and several suffered from mental illnesses. Her parents were inaccessible and powerless, resulting in profound emotional neglect and a highly anxious environment. Rachel's response, besides trying to be invisible, was to be the one who would care for and suffer with the others. Without even the most elementary consistent mirroring, that admiring reflection in the mother's face that welcomes the child to its life, or the presence of appropriately strong models to idealize and align herself with, she abandoned her true self, her center of initiative and self-knowledge, denying its feelings, needs and rights, in order to exist for others.

While this being for others made her excruciatingly sensitive to the needs and pain of others, she was rarely ever able to trust anyone with her own needs in a mutually negotiated fashion. She was simultaneously closed-off and unknown and highly vulnerable to being disappointed by others. Her own estrangement from herself, brought on by the chronically faulty responses of her care-giving milieu, led to the belief that she could never be known by another. To be in relationship meant to give up self, to never own anything, to give away whatever she had before it was taken. Her resulting relational failures and ambivalence toward the therapeutic bond, chock full of parental transferences, brought years of anguish for both of us in the struggle for trust.

Treatment Process

Through the years, many different interventions, both secular and religious, were tried in order to break through the depression and to set Rachel free to know and own herself and her life. Since we shared a similar faith perspective, this included different types of inner healing and generational prayer, from myself and others. Medications seemed to allow for some ground to be gained, but Rachel's overall experience was that it hurt to be alive.

Maintaining my faith and hope in the midst of such apparent therapeutic failure, while subject to Rachel's understandable episodes of rage, disappointment, and accusations, was obviously a struggle. I would question my own reality-testing, adequacy as a therapist, and countertransference issues, and seek consultation. But, at the same time, I always saw life and healing occurring within her. While I was open to helping her process the possibility that she should terminate or seek other therapy, I also recognized the essential nature of the attachment that Rachel had with me, anxious and ambivalent though it was. That bond included her recognition of my suffering with her and our joint acceptance of the challenge that her suffering was to our understanding of God and his ways. Her chronic emotional pain demanded that we take a contemplative stance - all our actions had failed! - and just be together and let God be God.

Present Goals

In the past year, Rachel's increasing ability to maintain trust in me, in God's faithful love for her, and in a compassionate connectedness with her self, has opened up the possibility of more consistent and focused prayer interventions. The goals have been:
1. to reduce her anxiety and depression, allowing fuller functioning in her life;
2. to increase her individuation from her family and her freedom to respond to them in new ways;
3. to increase her capacity to relate to others from a position of safety;
4. to allow her to bond with and own her core self so that she might claim and enjoy her life.

Current Process

A typical session begins with Rachel speaking for a long time and my saying very little. I have learned to be silent and to allow her to move into her interior, seeking the truth of her being at that moment and gaining comfort at being present to herself and to me. I work very hard to stay with her and to gently check out my understandings of what she is expressing. Any empathic break brings on distress and demands immediate repair. She is gifted in her ability to identify her internal processes and, as she speaks, an issue or theme emerges, directing further conversation and, ultimately, prayer.

During the prayer, I will often receive visual images which I share with Rachel and to which she may add or fine-tune. The image is a way of quickly mapping out a situation and inviting God's intervention, freeing Rachel of her old repetitive responses. For example, during a time of distress regarding her family's hold on her, I saw her in a raft, shoving off from shore, where they all remained in their misery. It was very difficult for her to leave them behind and she needed to know that not only was that okay, but that it was what the Lord required. She had to see that he was their God, too. Once she accepted this, the image brought her great relief and she was able to return to it while in actual situations with her family. Further meditations of her own enhanced the image. Jesus has joined her on the boat and together they now explore the darkness that has shrouded her life.

Outcome

The prayer and faith imagery have provided comfort and relief for Rachel on both an immediate and a long-term basis. They have offered her a kind of spiritual allegory in which she is able to recognize herself, owning and participating in the freeing reality of her relationships with Jesus and with me and with her true self, abandoned so long ago. Calling upon this eternal reality calms and centers her and coheses and enlivens her self, allowing her to be strengthened for her life struggles. As such, the image itself has become a selfobject experience, a representation of her true, safe, loved self with the power to make her whole.

It is Rachel's belief that our mutual faith has allowed her to endure. She now finds herself acceptable to the Lord and in total confidence of his love. She is increasingly strong and at ease in her boundary-setting, which is the key to the next step of keeping herself safe enough to risk relationship.

Discussion

It is clear to me that the methodology which I have put forth has largely been designed by Rachel herself. Just as empathic mothering is a two-way process, with the infant as a source of initiative, determining the pattern of responsiveness, so, too, is relational therapy. It is a reflection of our caring and compassionate God, respecting our freedom and inviting us to become co-creators in the cosmic dance. To enter into such a challenging relationship with less than a humble view toward mutual encounter and exploration of the great questions of existence would doom any attempt at healing.

There are many worthy ways to analyze human data and to practice the art of psychotherapy. There are also many ways to practice Christian therapy. The therapist's personality type and areas of giftedness and limitation, as well as her theological and psychological understandings, will help determine the ultimate expression of her practice. But the other major factor is the seeker herself: the personality, disorder, and spirituality of the hurting person impacts powerfully on the parameters of our healing art.

References

Bowen, M. (1978). *Family Therapy in Clinical Practice*. New York: Jason Aronson.

Elson, M. (1986). *Self Psychology in Clinical Social Work*. New York: W.W. Norton & Company.

Erikson, E. (1994). *Identity and the Life Cycle*. W.W. Norton & Company.

Jordan, J.V., Kaplan, A.G., Miller, J.B., Stiver, I.P. and Surrey, J.L. (1991). *Women's Growth in Connection*. New York: The Guilford Press.

Kohut, H. (1976). *The Restoration of the Self*. New York: International Universities Press.

Wolf, E.S. (1988). *Treating the Self*. New York: The Guilford Press.

Chapter 11

The Miracle of Therapy: Finding a New Way of Being*

Georgiana G. Rodiger, Ph.D.
69 North Catalina Ave.
Pasadena, CA 91106

Practitioner

Georgiana G. Rodiger, Ph.D. received her M.A. in Theology with an emphasis in marriage, family and child counseling from Fuller Theological Seminary and her Ph.D. in Clinical Psychology from the Fuller Graduate School of Psychology. Presently she is head of the Georgiana Rodiger Center, a nonprofit corporation, and has been previously associated with the Pasadena Community Counseling Center and the psychiatric division of Children's Hospital in Los Angeles.

Journey of Integration

Georgiana was privileged to attend a seminary that realized the necessity for Christians to understand human behavior and learn how to set captives free from psychological bondage. Fuller Theological Seminary in Pasadena, California, established a School of Psychology, and a Marriage, Family, and Child Counseling Program in the late 1960s, despite violent disagreement from some of Fuller's conservative supporters. It was a bold move; opposition ran high. These upstarts pressed on bravely into new territory, establishing the finest school in the world for educating Christian mental health professionals.

As a student at Fuller from 1973 to 1980, Georgiana was deeply moved by being part of the intensive effort the Seminary expended in studying the integration of theological and behavioral truths. Adhering strictly to the Scriptures, the students and faculty hammered out a Christian understanding of psychological discoveries. Students and faculty discussed every kind of intra-psychic and external problem possible on life's journey, exploring ways to give sight to the blind and freedom to the captive. She found this a joyous time - praying and studying with bright men and women who loved the Lord!

Context

The man described in this paper was seen at the Rodiger Center, where

---

* Reprinted from Rodiger, G. (1989). *The Miracle of Therapy*. Dallas, TX: Word Publishing.

Georgiana Rodiger supervises trainees and interns from masters and doctoral programs. At the Center therapists use a variety of therapies (cognitive-behavioral, humanistic, dynamic, existential, etc.), selecting the ones most appropriate for each client/patient.

Many of the clients seen at the Rodiger Center are not Christians. It is the ethical responsibility of therapists at the Center to work with clients within the parameters of their value systems, and not to try to convert them to the therapist's values and beliefs. Therapists at the Center are absolutely forbidden to evangelize those who come to the Center for therapy. It would be unethical to do so. Center therapists use Christian terminology with those who speak that language, secular psychological terminology with others. All value systems are honored as part of the growth of the client.

Theory/Theology
For God did not give us a spirit of fear, but a spirit of power, of love and of self-control" (2 Timothy 1:7).

This paper is excerpted from the author's book *The Miracle of Therapy* (Rodiger, 1989). Dr. Rodiger has chosen this title because in therapy miracles occur. A miracle is an extra-ordinary happening, not explicable through rational, scientific cause-and-effect reasoning. A miracle is a change we couldn't expect because it is out of the ordinary. We may hope for a miracle or even claim a miracle, as in declaring that a paralyzed child will walk, but it is always a great mystery as to when and where it will be effected. Miracles in therapy are also a great mystery because they require a number of unknown variables in the interaction between the patient and the therapist.

The constant is that God always wants to heal. His Son came among us healing all those around Him of diverse mental and physical ills. God has promised to be in our midst when "two or three come together in (His) name" (Matthew 1&20). He longs to bring us to maturity (Ephesians 4:13), to transform our minds into Christ's mind (Romans 12:2).

Therapy is an adventure in healing; recovery comes from insights, changed feelings and new behaviors. Without God's Living Power transmitted through the therapeutic hour and during the rest of the week, a patient cannot change from habitual ways of perceiving, feeling and behaving. Freed from the spirit of fear a client gains power, the ability to love and be loved and a sound mind because God wills the miracle of transformation. The old man dies as the new creation in Christ (2 Corinthians 5:17) is born. To Him be the glory!

Life is a school of hard knocks to bring us to a realization of the only possession of true value - a relationship with God. Daily we are given opportunities to practice self-control, patience, sweet spiritedness in the face of adversity, persistence despite failures, kindness and meekness. Despite our best efforts to manage life effectively—something external or internal often throws us off balance.

We can all remember disappointments and hurts. For some, getting through each day is very difficult. The job, the family, the adult toys, even recreational activities cease to give pleasure. Others have suffered a grievous loss through death, divorce, a diagnosis of progressive illness, a move away from loved ones, or sudden unemployment.

No matter how hard we try, we run into brick walls. Carefully picking ourselves up, checking for broken bones, dusting ourselves off, we vow we'll never let that catastrophe overtake us again. Diligently we plan for future success, trying to anticipate impediments along the way. All goes well for awhile and we settle into self-satisfaction. We've figured out how to live. We don't need anyone's help. Those poor slobs who keep getting into difficulties, we think to ourselves, should seek our advice on parenting, interpersonal relationships, employment, self-management and the spiritual life.

Then, when we least expect it, the brick wall again rises in our own path. We smash into it! Smug belief in the capacity to manage ourselves lies in the dust around us. "Unfair!" we shout. "We haven't done anything to deserve this setback," we complain. "Why did I get cancer? I'm too young to die," we moan. "My child can't be flunking first grade!" "My boss couldn't be firing me!" "It's not right!" "God must be asleep, letting all these bad things happen to me!"

We moan and groan and complain because life doesn't work out the way we expect. We feel cheated, unhappy, unappreciated; we begin to lose our motivation to keep going. Depression and bitterness often are the aftermath of repeated wall bumping. It gets harder and harder to hope things will work out. Even faith in God is often shaken. He should have kept the children from getting hurt in the automobile accident. He should have rewarded faithful service on the job with a promotion instead of a layoff.

Very few people come into therapy just to learn about themselves or examine their lives. Some do and find that therapy is a more exciting and rewarding exploration than a trip around the world. Investigating the unknown parts of ourselves, called the unconscious, is like entering a great underground cave full of hidden treasures. The flashlight of insight illuminates sparkling gems, secret passages, small lakes, soaring chambers, hidden wonders. Many people continue in therapy for the excitement of ongoing growth, but they start because they've hit a wall.

The Last Resort

Most individuals seeking therapy want change. The problems that brought them to a mental health professional make life uncomfortable, if not unbearable. The therapist is a last resort; most people would prefer to visit the dentist. To admit we have a problem managing our lives is very humiliating. Desire for relief from symptoms is the spur that pushes a client into making the first call. Then, the appointment made, anxiety increases until, with sweating palms and pounding heart, the moment of first contact arrives. Hope alternates with doubt as the conversation begins. *Can this doctor really help me? Will I be able to explain clearly what's bothering me? Will he think I'm stupid because I haven't been able to think through a solution? Will he feel I'm foolish for not having been able to change my behavior? Will I have to share embarrassing details about my life? Will the doctor lecture, as some of my friends have lectured, or give advice I can't seem to use? Will he be shocked by what I have done or how* I *think?*

These, and many other questions, rush frantically through a client's mind as he presents himself for therapy. It takes real courage to keep that first appointment, as anyone who has taken this step knows. And it costs real money, hard-earned dollars. Somehow, paying for talking seems unfair!

We all talk to each other all the time. Why does talking to this stranger cost an arm and a leg? Does he really know how to deal with my kind of trouble? Maybe I'm just wasting my time and money. It's hard to schedule in weekly appointments; my time is already squeezed between work and family responsibilities. Is my life so uncomfortable or so unfulfilled that I must move into the great unknown? What skills do I need to be a good client? What stress or discomfort will I undergo? Will I emerge with all my abilities intact? Is the expense and the risk really worth it? I've listened to the tales of those who have gone through therapy, and I've read books about the process. But can I trust those others? Would my experience be comparable? Have I chosen the right therapist for my kind of problem?

There are many different kinds of therapists and a variety of systems. In dentistry, at least, presumably filling a cavity is filling a cavity. Any trained, licensed dentist can diagnose and treat a sore tooth. However, unraveling the mysteries of human behavior is a far more complex business. Many paths are available; many guides promise health and comfort.

Gurus shout from radios and television sets: "I know how to make you happy, wealthy, thin, sexual, successful." Magazines contain articles about problems and how to solve them according to an expert in the field of mental health. Books filled with promises come out daily and are popular best sellers. Many of them denigrate other systems' ideas and interventions.

It is a bewildering maze. Dire consequences are foretold for the unwary who trust in the wrong therapist. Everyone hears of clients who have been in treatment for years, spending thousands of dollars, and are worse off than they were before they began. Psychiatric horror stories get big headlines suggesting futility, if not danger, for those who embark upon the adventure of psychological growth.

Church-centered Terror

For Christians, it's even worse. Some churches teach that healing for mental pain is appropriately sought only through prayer, fasting and the laying on of hands. To go into therapy is considered sinful, a cause for chastisement from the pastor and embarrassment within the congregation. If a person seeks professional mental help, he may be asked to resign his membership.

John came into therapy with pressures and beliefs like these. He called me because his physician suggested he consult a psychologist to alleviate recurrent severe headaches. Elaborate medical tests had ascertained that nothing was physically wrong, suggesting a psychological cause for his pain. John's ability to work was suffering, as well as his capacity to meet the needs of his wife and children.

Seldom have I seen a more terrified man. He had insisted on an appointment after dark and told me he would pay in cash. When he scheduled the appointment, he asked me not to record his name in my book, just his initials, and he questioned whether I needed to jot down information. I assured him I would honor his requests. Then he asked if I knew anyone from a particular church fifty miles away from my office. Reassured by my negative response, John appeared at the appointed hour, looking furtively around at others in the waiting room. As I ushered him into my office, he pressed cash into my hand and told me he had parked his car several blocks away. He apologized for these elaborate precautions, explaining a story now familiar to me about a pastor who forbade his flock to seek psychological counsel on pain of hellfire preceded by excommunication.

Beliefs such as "Psychology is of the Devil; marriage and family counselors deliberately lead people away from God's Word; therapists invade your thinking as the Devil invaded Eve's thinking; God is sufficient for all our needs without any interventions except prayer and fasting!" thundered from the pulpit of John's church every Sunday morning.

I asked John if his pastor was equally opposed to medical consultations or surgical interventions. Nervously, he replied that his pastor believed God used those doctors when necessary for healing; only mental health professionals were identified as belonging to the Prince of Darkness. He was frankly terrified of the magical power he believed I possessed; but he was equally terrified of the imminent loss of his ability to support his family if the headaches persisted.

When John nervously sought my help, I was able to assure him that I was not in the employ of Satan, nor did I have magical powers. Mental health professionals are guides, trained to bring seekers through the wilderness. With the help of the Holy Spirit, I could ascertain if there were psychological reasons for John's problems. We know the language of the unconscious, and how to help him find more adequate tools to manage himself in daily living and stress-filled situations. I wouldn't take control of his life (God is our Lord and Master) or teach him anything that was not scripturally based.

John was astonished. He asked how a pastor so learned and sound in other matters could be misinformed about therapy. I replied, "To the best of my understanding, it is because Freud thought God was a projection of the unconscious, and Watson believed that scientific methodology required leaving the unmeasurable out of the equation. Older pastors may not have been exposed to the writings of Christian psychologists and psychologically knowledgeable Christians."

Junior

I call the part of ourselves which controls most of our thoughts, feelings and behaviors *Junior*, or *the unconscious*. No one who is comfortable with all his feelings and behaviors comes to talk to a therapist. I understand that my task is to discover the way a client's Junior sabotages his good intentions and desired thoughts. Saint Paul said, "I do not understand what I do. For what I want to do, I do not do, but what I hate I do" (Romans 7:15).

We study Junior's values, beliefs, and desires through talking about what the client has done during the week, how he felt and what he dreamed. A good client learns to talk about his daily life, and to notice unusual thoughts, feelings, and actions. He remembers dreams. As we carefully scrutinize this material, the client and I become more and more aware of the *little one* inside. Junior is often no more than two or three years old. If you think about the two-year-olds you have known, it becomes obvious why bad habits and thought patterns are hard to break. Two-year-olds are opinionated, stubborn, oppositional, selfish and intensely involved with their feelings. When angry, they have temper tantrums; when pleased, they are filled with hugs and kisses.

By thirty-six months of age, all of us have learned a great deal about the nature of reality and interpersonal relationships. If our mothers have been available to us for most of every day and our households relatively free from tension, we feel comfortable in the world and in relationships. A well-nurtured three-year-old likes himself so well he is convinced others should do things his way. He has learned the rules about eating, bedtime, bath, car trips, shopping, gifts, Sunday school, grandparents, toys, parks, animals, television, swimming pools, flowers, breakable objects, knives, etc. He knows he is loved unequivocally. The love God has for people is transmitted to the young child through the unconditional affection of his parents. He is able to stand up to giants (adults) and say, "No, not those jammies," "Give me a lollipop," "I hate you; you're a bad mommy," and "I love you."

Securely grounded, the child can attend to learning how objects and relationships function in the world. He feels the difference between throwing a glass or a ball, or between hugging a cat or a snail. He experiences hitting a parent or biting another child. He observes the relationships between parents and children, lovers, siblings, pastors and people, grandparents, dogs and postmen. If the child continues to be in a safe environment with loving adults, he learns by watching and experimenting with the way the world works; he begins to understand people's feelings. He enjoys his capacities and accepts his failings. Learning in school and on the playground comes easily because his anxiety is minimal.

For most of the people we see in therapy the preceding was not the scenario. When they were little, their parents were stressed because of family, financial, or personal problems. Their homes were full of tension or fighting. Sometimes they were severely scolded for misusing or breaking objects, often producing in the adult a timid approach to experiences in the world. Frequently they were left for long periods with strangers, babysitters, or daycare workers, resulting in abandonment fears and disturbed love relationships as adults. Buried deep inside many of us, carefully shielded from the conscious mind, is a loving, raging infant with faulty perceptions about the true nature of reality. The task of the therapist is to be a guide for the client, encouraging each step, as he explores infantile feelings and beliefs.

There are expected thrills and obstacles for the therapeutic voyager. Junior's opinions and desires are often not acceptable to the adult person sitting before me so the patient blocks them out of his awareness. For example, the child who substituted cookies for her absent mother, filling herself with sweets to fill the aching void, may find dieting difficult as an adult despite extensive nutritional information. The reason she cannot lose weight is centered much more in Junior's needs that produce compulsive overeating, than in her adult decisions.

The man who quits his job each time he begins to be promoted and paid adequately may be driven by an unconscious fear of losing his dad if he achieves success, due to a faulty connection between his academic success in kindergarten and his parents' divorce. We know his competence did not cause the marital breakup, but his *little mind* put two and two together and came up with five.

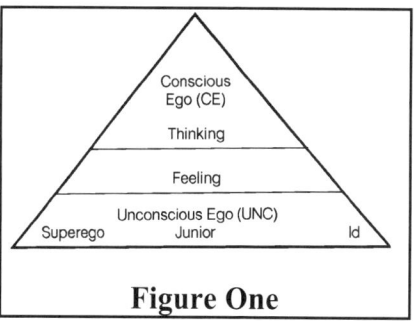

Journeying together, the patient and the clinician explore the unconscious. When familiar landmarks appear, they can understand why the woman eats or the man quits. He or she can then learn other ways to deal with the conflict arising from early experiences.

Figure One

(Triangle diagram: Conscious Ego (CE) / Thinking / Feeling / Unconscious Ego (UNC) Junior; Superego on left, Id on right)

Understanding Personalities

A further word about the makeup of human personality might be in order as a point of reference for subsequent discussions. Imagine, if you will, a triangle pointing upward (See Figure One). Then imagine drawing two horizontal lines through the center of the triangle. These lines represent the repression barrier. In it are the ego defenses. Label the upper line *thinking* and the lower line *feeling*. In the top point of the triangle write *Conscious Ego* (CE). Below the two lines write *Unconscious Ego* (UNC) or *Junior*. *Superego* and *Id* go in the left and right lower corners respectively.

Now picture, if you will, a battle going on most of the time between the superego and the id in the bottom of our triangle. The id says, "I want to eat a dozen donuts"; and the superego says, "You'll get fat." The id says, "I want to play all day"; the superego says, "you have to support your family." The conscious ego's job (the top of the triangle) is to deal with the world and get on with daily living. He cannot spend time and energy attending to the battle; he blocks it out of his mind. This is called *repression*. He pushes it down below the two lines and is unaware it is going on at all. Some people are more able to do this than others. Psychotics, so-called crazy people, can't do it at all; others have major difficulties repressing uncomfortable material.

Repression is a defense. It defends the person from having to think about (cognition) or feel (affect) the battle between the superego and the id. There are a number of other defenses. For example, instead of feeling rage at a mother who wasn't really there for Junior, a woman might get very involved in *La Leche League*, teaching new mothers to be available to their infants through long-term breastfeeding. That's the defense of *sublimation*. Or she might become a research psychologist and study the bonding needs of infants, including hours of observations on mother-baby interactions. That is the defense of *intellectualiza*tion, defending against the pain of longing for mother by understanding the dyadic (bonding) relationship.

Rather than stand the distress of hearing parents' arguing all the time, a child might develop asthma. Each asthmatic attack would stop the fights as both parents rush to help their suffocating youngster. Careful tracking by a trained specialist who links the asthma attacks with family fights might indicate a psychological as well as a physical origin. This is the defense of *somatization.*

Other defenses will be discussed in the case history. Of course, my simplistic model of a human being as a triangle is only a tool to help us understand unconscious conflicts and defenses. The battle between our basic wishes for immediate comfort and our parents', teachers', or bosses' voices within us saying, "Get to work," "You'll get fat," "Save for tomorrow," "Be kind," and many other injunctions never stops during our lifetime. We can use more sophisticated defenses once we have insight into why we do what we do, but we can never quiet the inner battle completely.

Into this lifelong task our God comes, bringing forgiveness and the peace that passes understanding. What that means is that His peace is able to quiet the internal wrangling as He calmed the storm. He made us and lived here, in the person of Jesus, so He knows what we experience. He is our Comforter, the Rock upon which we stand.

The Therapist's Perspective and Methodology

As a Christian therapist, I know that our God reigns. He has dominion over all conflict and darkness; His light illumines our struggles; His Word informs our words. I know the darkest hour comes just before the dawn. The worst pain can be borne by those formed in God's image and likeness; the cruelest conflicts can be resolved because Jesus is the Great Mediator. As a guide through the wilderness of each person's unique history and problems, I know that the Land of Milk and Honey can be reached by those who go forward despite intra-psychic pain and fear. It can be uncomfortable to search our unconscious and find our inappropriate defenses. The reward is entering into the Promised Land.

Therapists give new perspectives, just as God called people throughout the Scriptures to see events in a new way. Abraham's descendants are numbered as the stars because of his obedience, not because of the miracle of Isaac's birth to a ninety-year-old woman. If Abraham had believed Isaac was the key to the promise, he would never have prepared to sacrifice him. Moses knew a Land of Milk and Honey was awaiting the children of Israel. If he had lost faith as the months became years, the people would have been without a guide. Even his relative and spokesman before the Pharaoh, Aaron, succumbed to the people's fear, creating for them a golden calf, a false defense to be idolized.

If Jesus had accepted the prevailing cultural mores regarding the oldest son's duty to help his widowed mother with the younger children, the greatest life ever lived and most precious death ever died would not have happened. The Bible is a book of unexpected perspectives lived out in obedience to God's will, not man's common sense or institutionalized rules. Therapy must provide new visions of God's will in men's and women's lives.

Hitting the wall, I believe, is part of God's plan for our lives in this school of hard knocks called life. He doesn't send trouble, but He allows the Prince of Darkness to roam freely in the world, causing disharmony and tragedy. Flat in the dust we are given the opportunity with Job to say, "Even though He slay me, yet will I hope in him" (Job 13:15). Without hardships and disappointments, we become complacent, convinced we can manage our own lives. Only from our humble awareness of impotence can we truly cry, "Abba, Father."

Case Illustration
Synopsis
   Ray and his wife, Marge, had been devoted to the Lord all their lives. Their pastors suggested that steadfastness in daily prayer, reading of the Word, tithing, and church involvement would result in marital harmony and successful children. Ray became very depressed when his youngsters got into trouble. We resolved that crisis but three years later his wife asked him to move out. Ray became disoriented and extremely anxious away from his family. Instead of living alone, nursing his grievances, Ray decided to be a house parent in a home for disturbed youngsters. By giving them counsel and hope, he was transformed. Therapy allowed Ray to renew his covenanted relationship with Marge. God created in them "a pure heart" and renewed "a steadfast spirit" (Psalm 51:10).

Significant History and Presenting Issues
   I first met Ray and Marge to discuss their son's academic difficulties. Despite above average academic competence, Stan was flunking out of his senior year in high school. He refused to study, missed classes, and had disappeared for several days at a time. At home he was rude to his parents and mean to his little sister. Carol wasn't doing very well in the ninth grade either. She thought about clothes and boys exclusively it seemed. Ray and Marge were baffled as to why their children were turning out so badly. They had both spent a lot of time with them. They attended church regularly; the youngsters belonged to choir and youth groups. It was a puzzlement!
   Ray and Marge were attractive people in their early forties. He was a dentist. She went to work as an executive secretary in a medical firm after their daughter entered kindergarten. They both came from solid families of Scottish extraction. Her parents were farmers. His father was a grocer in Kansas. After the Second World War, they bought their present home in California.
   I hear this story over and over. Difficulties occur with the children even though the parents have conscientiously tried to do everything correctly. They had been to all the teachers' meetings, supervised homework, and made strict rules on the advice of a school psychologist, all to no avail. Both youngsters continued to act out. Stan wouldn't come home when he was told. Carol didn't help around the house. Stan was messy. Carol dressed very peculiarly, etc., etc., and so forth.

Therapeutic Process, Beginning
   The second time we talked together, I began to see that each parent was blaming the other. The father thought that the mother was too lenient; the mother thought that the father was too strict. They disagreed about money. Marge believed the children should be given money for various activities.

Ray believed they should earn it. They disagreed about recreation time. She believed the family should spend a lot of time together going places and doing things. He wanted to have his beloved wife to himself, on occasions.

Ray agreed Marge was a caring mother, but felt she was overly attentive to the children's desires and overly forgiving when they broke the rules. Marge thought Ray was stern and unsympathetic and didn't really understand the difficulties of being a teenager in today's world. They also disagreed about Marge's mother. Marge said the church taught she should see her mother every day, as the old lady was a widow with severe arthritis and failing eyesight. Ray believed she was spending far too much time attending to her mother.

I was able to help them be firm with Stan. They decided he could not live at home anymore if he didn't go to school regularly and maintain a C-average. I told Ray there were seven things that he and Marge should say to Stan and Carol every day and nothing else:

"Good morning."
"You look terrific!"
"Hope you have a good day."
"Here's a delicious breakfast for you."
"Dinner time."
"Hope you sleep well."
"Good night, my love."

They asked, "How will we get the chores done?"

"Write a note; stick it on the refrigerator listing all the chores you expect Stan and Carol to do each week. Allow them to decide when to do them."

"How can we be sure the dog gets fed?"

"If the dog isn't fed, take it to the animal shelter unless you want to feed it."

"How can we get their rooms tidied up?"

"If anything is out of place on Monday, hide it. Otherwise, ignore them."

Ray and Marge went home from that session and spelled out the new rules. The steady stream of criticism and advice stopped. Stan pulled himself together, worked very hard, and finished high school with a B- average. Carol took responsibility for her own schoolwork, limiting her social life voluntarily.

During further sessions, we rejoiced at the new tranquility and refined their reactions to annoying behavior. I spent a great deal of time encouraging Ray and Marge to trust their kids, urging them to start enjoying each other instead of worrying about Stan and Carol. I suggested they not talk about their youngsters at all, writing notes to each other if decisions had to be made. After several months their home had settled down so they decided to discontinue therapy.

Therapeutic Process, Midcourse

Three years later Ray called saying he needed to see me. I asked about the children and he reported they were doing very well in college. I was delighted. We set an appointment for the next week.

When he came in, Ray looked haggard and exhausted. A tall man, muscular from daily exercise, he was normally at the peak of health.

I asked, "What has happened?"

"My wife asked me to move out. We argue a lot. She has stopped wanting to make love. It's been hell."

This tragedy often happens. In systems' theory we learn that when people change, stresses and strains appear in other parts of the family. Until my previous intervention, the children had been the problem. Husband and wife were drawn together to help them. Daily conversations revolved around the latest misdemeanor, debating what they were going to do. When I forbade that kind of dialogue, encouraging them to begin enjoying each other, trouble started. The children ceased being the identified problem, the bad guys, and the parents discovered their interpersonal difficulties.

Ray explained, "There was more and more tension. Our sex life became almost nonexistent. I couldn't say anything without Marge yelling or crying. I don't know what's going on. Perhaps it's her menopause. It has been very uncomfortable around our home. She always talked about how her feelings were hurt because I didn't understand her or really care about the family. That's not true. I don't know what I did wrong. Last week Marge asked me to move out. She said she had been angry since the beginning of our marriage; she never really loved me. That hurts. She needs to get away from me to discover herself. I don't know what to do."

Ray was in real psychological danger. His identity was as Marge's husband and the children's father, the supporter of the family. The home, where he had spent many long hours fixing things, was his haven, his place of relaxation. Banned from the house, he was confused and anxious. In his small apartment he couldn't relax enough to cook, read, or watch television. Ray ate junk food, pacing about his apartment. Every night by three in the morning he was wide awake, having slept only a few hours.

Ray was seriously depressed. Every line in his body telegraphed unhappiness and abandonment. He told me at length about each situation where there had been a misunderstanding. He recited what she had said and what he had said and what other people had said. After two hours of listening, I finally remarked, "You'll get sick if you keep these thoughts going round and round in your mind."

"I know. It's awful. I can't stop thinking about my wife and the things we said to each other."

"The Bible tells us we have to forgive and go forward."

Angrily he replied, "That's easy to say but very difficult to do."

Calmly, "I know. I know. But you're poisoning yourself. I believe you'll be talking again within six months. In the meantime you need to stay steady, using this time to grow in your relationship with Christ."

"I know but it's lonely; I'm restless living by myself."

"Well, then, move in with my friend who runs a shelter for disturbed adolescents. They need another strong man around. You'd be able to teach them about the Lord."

His eyes brightened. "Would that be possible? I'd love to talk with those youngsters. Could I really be used to encourage them?"

"Of course. After work every day, you can go home to needy kids to play ball, eat dinner, hang out. On weekends you can teach them to ski, your favorite sport. They need your wisdom and counsel." Ray moved in the next week and enjoyed his time with the teenagers.

Marge wanted her freedom, and found Ray restrictive and non-empathic. She wasn't interested in joint counseling about their marriage. She longed to find her real self. Insisting she come in for weekly counseling on communication styles or family games was pointless. I knew that once the first flush of freedom wore off, Marge would begin to miss Ray's companionship. Because of the intricate interweaving of their lives for twenty-three years with friends, church, and children, separation would begin to feel like amputation.

My main fear was that another woman would come along and get her hooks into Ray before Marge had time to experience the loss. Though his depression would lift rapidly through pleasure in being admired, his mixed loyalties could be very hard to reconcile. Christians know marriage is a covenanted relationship. Given time, God always works on each heart for reconciliation. I discerned that they would come to their senses. In the meantime, Ray needed protection from aggressive women looking for a handsome, gentle man. In therapy we worked on learning to enjoy blessed singleness.

Commentary

Our Lord tells us that each man must learn to stand by himself. He made Peter leave his fishing and his wife, which gave his mother-in-law the vapors (Matthew 8:14). She was appalled that her son-in-law would follow a traveling teacher rather than support her and produce grandchildren as was customary in Israel. Jesus' willingness to separate spouses was hard to understand. "And everyone who has left houses or brothers or sisters or father or mother or wife or children or fields for my sake will receive a hundred times as much and will inherit eternal life" (Matthew 19:29).

In today's world being paired is more important than commitment to the living God. We are bombarded daily through the media with the idea that all single people yearn to be joined to somebody else. The old-fashioned concepts of blessed singleness and the joys of celibacy are considered foolish. It is a popular notion that one's mate is one's best friend, that a person can share anything with his significant other. Sex is the supreme event, signifying emotional and physical union.

Scripture indicates that the passionate, all-consuming involvement of the major figures in the Bible is their relationship with God. Some of them were married: Abraham, Isaac, Jacob, Moses, and Peter. But Jesus wasn't married and He didn't encourage His disciples to get married. He never said to any of His disciples, "Why don't you get engaged to that nice woman over there? You should have a family." He never said, "The family that prays together, stays together." Nor did He give insights into child rearing.

Of course, He honored marriage and forbade divorce. A stable, affectionate relationship between two people is the proper nurturing ground for children. An infant's long immaturity makes it very difficult for one person to meet all his emotional and physical needs. Single parenting can be done, as tragically we're seeing today in America, where many youngsters are being raised by one adult. But it certainly is not optimal. A child needs both a mother and a father, and, of course, Jesus knew that. But the raising of children wasn't a priority for the One who came to teach Kingdom living.

For centuries religious families gave their best, the strongest, brightest, and most creative child, to the church, and their second most capable son to support the country. Their third son devoted himself to business and supporting all the indigent relatives, carrying on the family lineage through children. A son or daughter dedicated to God, offering a lifetime of praise and service, was considered the highest good.

A mother was honored by her whole village if her child took holy orders. No need for grandchildren existed here; no sentimental Hallmark cards about grandmother were desired. Service of God was the most important calling. He was the One a person talked to when depressed and turned to for comfort in grief. God was the best companion in times of trouble and in times of joy, in times of celebration and in times of working.

This seems to be closer to Jesus' thinking than does the modern cult of finding a significant other, of having one's children take care of one's emotional needs, or worshiping grandchildren. Jesus came to tell us to walk the path rejoicing in the presence of God, talking with Him, laughing with Him, weeping with Him. Living that way, a person is not seduced by money or power or sexual attraction, nor dismayed by the disappointments and losses of this life. They are all relative; only God is absolute. As Kierkegaard said, "Render unto the relative, relatively and unto the absolute, absolutely." Jesus came to bring us the peace that passes understanding. Common sense doesn't understand how somebody can be peaceful in the midst of triumph and tragedy. But Christians know that life is a training school for our souls, a journey designed with mountains to climb, rivers to cross, and losses to endure. Joy comes in the midst of difficulties if our eyes are fixed on Christ.

Therapeutic Process, Continued
Ray was an enormous blessing to the young people. He counseled and played handball. As a good, strong man who loved the Lord passionately, he was the best possible witness for the disturbed kids with whom he lived.

Ray's depression lifted as he plunged into interacting. Ray was sad not to be with his wife and children, but he wasn't frantic anymore. He learned to enjoy his time alone, communing intimately with God. He no longer needed other people.

Therapeutic Process, Concluding Steps
After six months, Ray said, "My wife called and she wants me to come to dinner."

I exclaimed, "Wonderful! What fun!"

Suspiciously, "How should I handle it? I bet she wants money."

"Very carefully. Tell her that you love her and want to be with her. Do not bring up old resentments, gripes, and irritations."

Ray asked, "How will she know to stop doing all those distressing things?"

"She won't. But you've changed, and you'll find they don't bother you so much. You've mellowed, living with all those disturbed teenagers. You're not nearly as judgmental and rigid."

"You taught me to appreciate, admire, listen to, and enjoy the kids. Should I be with Marge the same way?"

"Yes, that's agape love, love without need."

"Okay," he remarked, "I'll try it." And so he did.

At our next session Ray looked radiant. He had increased his empathic listening skills attending to the young people. It was easy to take pleasure in his wife's recounting of various activities that she was enjoying. He liked looking at her, laughing with her, and using the "in" language they had developed during their marriage. When she brought up certain problems with the children that began to push his buttons, he remembered not to react. Smiling sweetly he'd ask, "Tell me how you feel about it. What do you think we ought to do?"

The reason Marge asked him to dinner was, indeed, to discuss money. Ray was very conservative when it came to dollars; he was a penny pincher. He wanted to save his substantial income for the education of his children and retirement. He had no interest in consumer goods. His wife, on the other hand, liked to keep a nice house and buy fashionable clothes. Money had always been a bone of contention between them. When finances came up at their reunion, Ray gripped the bottom of his chair to hold himself quiet. He listened calmly. When she asked for his opinion, he followed my instructions carefully. "Dear, I'll have to think about it. I don't know exactly what I want to do. Let me pray for twenty-four hours and I'll get back to you." She was visibly relieved that he hadn't become angry. They parted filled with new hope. Ray was elated because the evening had been enormously successful.

They continued to meet once a week for the next three months. He wouldn't fight. Every time she brought up an issue on which he had a strong opinion, he held his tongue. When she pressed him for an answer, he would say, "I have to pray about that."

Three months later Ray told me that Marge wanted to come to a session. I replied, "Fine, as long as you come, too." When they both came to my office, I was delighted to see her.

She said, "I am bewildered. I can't quite figure out whether this new behavior is for real. Will Ray continue to be able to listen without getting angry or is it some trick that you taught him to get back in my good graces?"

She talked at length about how she had agonized over asking him to move out. She loved him very much but found his rigid opinions and miserliness more than she could bear. He would storm around the house pointing out the sins and wickednesses of the children, neighbors, church people, and his office personnel.

"Since we have gotten back together again for dinner, Ray appears to be calm and cheerful. I know he doesn't always agree with me as to how to handle situations or money, but he doesn't lecture and make me feel like an ignoramus. I asked to see you because I want to know if this is going to last or will Ray become his old self when we move back together again?"

There were a number of different ways to answer. I could have replied, "You two will need a lot of marital counseling, communication training, and sexual therapy. We must explore unconscious conflicts so that you don't regress into bad patterns." Or, "If I were you, I'd be very careful because you can't teach an old dog new tricks. He'll probably revert when he's safely back in his own home."

I could have drawn up a behavioral program or tried to adjudicate their problems. I might have explained the games they played or their family systems.

Instead, God brought Joseph to my mind. So I talked about that very opinionated, self-righteous young man. The biblical narrative describes his flaunting the many-colored coat and his dreams about cattle and corn. Ray and Joseph had characteristics in common; they believed they were right until God humbled them.

God often allows a traumatic happening to produce change. In Joseph's case, after being sold into slavery in Egypt, he was jailed on false charges; in Ray's, it was being told by his beloved wife that he had to leave his home and family. God transformed both men from the inside out. They could not revert to their old arrogance. Ray's prayer over these long months to have the mind of Christ had been granted. "You can take him back with joy," I replied.

At home, Ray demonstrated a quiet humor, and an unwillingness to get drawn into arguments. Marge also changed. Issues which had seemed important faded in the harmony of their home. The effect on the children was dramatic. Instead of avoiding their parents, they began to come home from college for weekends to talk. They sought Ray's counsel, finding him available and wise. Marge delighted in their relationships and enjoyed the family get-togethers. The last I heard they were giving God the glory for their transformed lives.

Conclusion

God's healing power creates miracles. "Seek first His Kingdom and His righteousness, and all these things will be given to you as well" (Matthew 6:33). Ray's psyche was soaked in the Word; he had listened and read all his life. Despite difficulties in his childhood, which led to miserliness and rigidity, Ray yearned to have the mind of Christ.

He was not aware of his characterological disorder; it's very hard to know ourselves. For God to continue Ray's sanctification, Marge's heart was turned against him. Ray's judgments and penny pinching were the reasons given, but I suspect she lost her enthusiasm for being in his company. Little things he did annoyed her; mannerisms evoked rage. Marge never intended to feel irritable toward Ray. She began to feel suffocated in their relationship. I believe God arranged these occurrences so that they could become mature, "attaining to the whole measure of the fullness of Christ" (Ephesians 4:13).

They both grew up. With Ray gone from the house, Marge was able to experience herself and sort out her internal feelings from her reactions to Ray. She became more open to him, able to forgive as the weeks lengthened into months. Ray's rigid beliefs had been jolted repeatedly living with disturbed young adults. As he listened to them talk, trying to provide help and comfort, his life with Marge looked very blessed in hindsight. He empathized with his own children, realizing they had been through identity crises he hadn't understood at the time.

As a result of insights gained in therapy, Ray became less authoritarian. Initially, he was a poor candidate for counseling because he didn't think anything was wrong with him. He knew right from wrong and believed a man should teach his family. It was good stewardship to be very careful with money. I could have told him in our first session that he needed more empathy for others' opinions, but he wouldn't have been able to make that insight operational in his life. God provided the young adults for his growth. They shared themselves with him and he grew to love those very unlike himself. Ray's giving of himself, instead of obsessing about Marge's unfairness, provided the plowed field into which seeds of self-knowledge could be sown in therapy.

Discussion: Becoming Citizens of the Kingdom
The infinite variety of human experiences is God's way of making us citizens of the kingdom. To transform us into disciples, we have to be derailed from our habitual ways of being. Peter, Andrew, James, and John gave up their nets to beg for daily bread. Mr. and Mrs. Zebedee lost the earning power of their strong sons in a day when sons were the only social security and retirement plan. Saul lost his political influence, his rabbinical prestige, and his capacity to earn enough to live a comfortable life when he became the apostle Paul. At his brain power level, with his advanced degrees, tent making was a real occupational loss of status. He didn't come from a family of tent makers; he never envisioned he'd work with his hands. New wine is not put in old wineskins (Matthew 9:17).

I am always amazed that Christians are so surprised when their lives go off-track. Jesus began His ministry by leaving Nazareth. His mother needed His carpentry to support the younger children; she needed His emotional help to raise the four little kids. His school friends, the boys He coached in ball games, the students He taught at the synagogue, the old ladies He helped with chores around their homes - all of them depended on Him. He just walked away. People say, "But He was God." Of course, He was God. He took on human flesh and became a man to show us how to live. "He was in the world, and though the world was made through Him, the world did not recognize Him" (John 1:10-11), because its people were too stuck on their familiar tracks.

"The world is too much with us late and soon. Getting and spending we lay waste our powers. Little we know of nature that is ours." (In this poem, nature means God's creation.) Wordsworth goes on to say, "Oh God, I'd rather be a pagan suckled on a creed outworn, so might I, standing on this pleasant lea, have glimpses that would make me less forlorn."

Forlorn we are in this age of anxiety. We cannot see God's hand molding us into appropriate vessels for His Holy Spirit. "We are poor little lambs who have lost our way, baa, baa, baa. We are poor little sheep who have gone astray baa, baa, baa ... God have mercy on such as we, baa, baa, baa!" *(Whiffenpoof* song, Yale University)

What is "the poor little lamb's" way? Jesus is the "way, the truth, and the life" (John 14:6). What is the plan of creation? Jesus came to show us how to live. If His life jumped out of habitual tracks, why are we so surprised when our lives are turned upside down?

Unfortunately, comfort and predictability have been promised to faithful churchgoers, instead of the pilgrim's way that ends with a cross. Health and wealth, prosperity theology, leads to damnation. Apostate churches prioritize social activities and good deeds, forgetting that Jesus said our main concern must be a right relationship with God. Works flow out of transformed lives filled with the Holy Spirit.

"Therefore if any man be in Christ, he is a new creature: old things are passed away, behold, all things are become new" (2 Corinthians 5:17).

References

Anonymous. *Prayer of a Confederate Soldier.*

Bowen, M. (1978). *Family Therapy in Clinical Practice.* New York: Jason Aronson.

Freud, S. (1961). "The ego and the id and other works." In *The Standard Edition of the Complete Psychological Works of Sigmund Freud, Volume XIX (1923-1925)* [Strachey, J., trans. & ed.]. London: Hogarth Press and The Institute of Psycho-Analysis.

Freud, S. (1963). "Introductory lectures on psycho-analysis (Parts I and II)." In *The Standard Edition of the Complete Psychological Works of Sigmund Freud, Volume XV (1915-1916).* [Strachey, J., trans. & ed.]. London: Hogarth Press and The Institute of Psycho-Analysis.

Freud, S. (1963). "Introductory lectures on psycho-analysis (Part III)." In *The Standard Edition of the Complete Psychological Works of Sigmund Freud, Volume XVI (1916-1917).* [Strachey, J., trans. & ed.]. London: Hogarth Press and The Institute of Psycho-Analysis.

Holy Bible: King James Version. (1949). Glasgow: William Collins, Sons and Company, Ltd., 1949; Philadelphia: The Westminister Book Stores.

Jones, Warren L. (1988). Personal communication, an unpublished manuscript. Pasadena, California.

Kierkegaard, Soren. (1941, 1951). *Fear and Trembling and The Sickness Unto Death* (Lowrie, W. trans.). Princeton, NJ: Princeton University Press.

Kierkegaard, Soren. (1944, 1957). *The Concept of Dread* (Lowrie, W. trans.). Princeton, NJ: Princeton University Press.

Klein, M. (1948). "The development of the child" (1921). In *Contributions to Psychoanalysis, 1921-1945.* London: Hogarth Press.

Kohut, H. (1971). *The Analysis of the Self.* New York: International Universities Press.

Kohut, H. (1977). *The Restoration of the Self.* New York: International

Universities Press.

Mahler, M. (1968). *On Human Symbiosis and the Vicissitudes of Individuation, Vol. I: Infantile Psychosis*. New York: International Universities Press.

Minuchin, S. (1974). *Families and Family Therapy*. Cambridge: Harvard University Press.

Rogers, C. (1961). *Client-Centered Therapy*. Boston: Houghton Mifflin.

Sullivan, H.S. (1953). *Interpersonal Theory of Psychiatry*. New York: Norton.

Thompson Chain-Reference Bible: New International Version. (1983). Indianapolis, IN: B.B. Kirkbride Bible Company, Inc. & Grand Rapids: The Zondervan Corporation.

Winnicott, D.W. (1964). *The Child, the Family, and the Outside World*. New York: Penguin Books.

Winnicott, D.W. (1965). *The Maturational Processes and the Facilitating Environment: Studies in the Theory of Emotional Development*. New York: International Universities Press.

Whitaker, C.A. and Napier, A.Y. (1978). *The Family Crucible*. New York: Harper and Row.

Wordsworth, W. (1969). "The world is too much with us." In *Poems of William Wordsworth*. Wimbish Village near Saffron Walden/Essex, England: Collection Chosen & Published by Geoffrey Parker.

Key Words

1. *Abandonment Anxiety/Abandonment Fear*: Mixed feelings of dread and apprehensions that one will ultimately be deserted by those one loves and/or attempts to love, but without a specific current cause for this fear. Typically, such persons have experienced significant losses and/or separations from parents and/or significant others during infancy or childhood.
2. *Actualize*: See Self-Actualization
3. *Adult*: The term employed by Eric Berne to describe that consistent pattern of feeling, experience, and behavior of an individual (i.e., ego state) that is "oriented toward objective, autonomous data-processing and probability estimating" (Berne, 1966, p. 36).
4. *Affect*: "A broad class of mental processes, including feeling, emotion, moods, and temperament" (Chaplin, 1975, p. 14).
5. *Anxiety*: "An affect that differs from other affects in its specific unpleasurable characteristics. Anxiety consists of a somatic, physiological side (disturbed breathing, increased heart activity, vasomotor changes, musculoskeletal disturbances such as trembling or paralysis, increased sweating, etc.) and of a psychological side …. Fear is a reaction to a real

or threatened danger, while anxiety is more typically a reaction to an unreal or imagined danger" (Campbell, 1981, pp.41-42).
6. *Bonding*: The term used by Winnicott et al to describe the crucial relationship between the mother and her infant consisting of accurate empathic nonverbal communication developed through touching, holding, staring at each other, imitation, and responsive interactions. Some researchers feel bonding is a biological need, like eating and breathing.
7. *Conflict*: "The simultaneous occurrence of two or more mutually antagonistic impulses or motives" (Chaplain, 1975, p. 109).
8. *Defense Mechanism*: "Any behavior pattern which protects the psyche from anxiety, shame, or guilt. Some common defense mechanism are: repression, regression, projection, identification, fantasy, compensation, sublimation, reaction-formation, and aggression" (Chaplin, 1975, p. 131).
9. *Depression*: "In the normal individual, a state of despondency characterized by feelings of inadequacy, lowered activity, and pessimism about the future. In pathological cases, an extreme state of unresponsiveness to stimuli, together with self-depreciation, delusions of inadequacy, and hopelessness" (Chaplin, 1975, p. 135).
10. *Dyadic Intimacy/Dyadic Relationship:* see also Bonding. An intimate relationship between two persons.
11. *Dynamic Problems:* Conflicts of an unconscious nature that cause maladaptive behaviors in an individual.
12. *Ego:* "One of the three agencies which compose the structure of the psyche …. The ego is the central agency of the personality, whose task is to mediate the conflicting demands of the superego, the id and those of external reality …. The ego employs censorship to modify the instinctual drives and signals anxiety when the contents of the id threaten to overwhelm it, whilst its own defense mechanisms protect it from threat from the external world …. According to Freud, the ego develops gradually out of the id through having to adapt to the demands of external reality. It is built up through the introjection of part objects and object relations. Melanie Klein, however, conceives of the ego as existing embryonically from birth and of being capable of distinguishing the self from the object. And so, from the beginning it uses primitive defense mechanisms such as splitting and projection" (Walrond-Skinner, 1986, p. 108).
13. *Empathy:* "Putting oneself into the psychological frame of reference of another, so that the other person's thinking, feeling, and acting are understood and, to some extent predictable. Carl Rogers defines empathy as the ability to accompany another wherever the other person's feelings lead him, no matter how strong, deep, destructive, or abnormal they may seem" (Campbell, 1981, p. 215).

14. *Family Dynamics/Family System:* The manner in which a family system is interrelated and how it interacts. A change in one part of the family system will cause changes in other parts of the family system.
15. *Id:* One of the three agencies which between them compose the structure of the psyche, according to psychoanalytic theory. The id represents the major portion of the unconscious, although it is not co-terminus with it, since both the ego and the superego have unconscious aspects .... Freud (Freud, S. 'The ego and the id'; *Standard Edition*, vol. 19, 1923, Hogarth Press. London) viewed the id as 'a chaos ... filled with energy reaching it from the instincts. It has no organization, produces no collective will but only a striving to bring about the satisfaction of instinctual needs subject to the observance of the pleasure principle.' In its lack of organization and its complete unconsciousness it stands in contrast to both the ego and the superego .... Haman (Haman, A. 'What do we mean by id?'; *J. of Am. Psychoanalytic Assoc.*, 1969, vol. 17, pp. 353-380) suggests that the id is best understood as a way of acting that conforms to the infantile mode – irrational, unrestrained and heedless of consequences or contradictions. Such spontaneous action can either be aggressively egocentric or creatively part of lateral thinking and hence independent and novel in its results" (Walrond-Skinner, 1986, pp. 174-175).
16. *Intellectualization (an ego defense):* A defense mechanism in which a person analyzes a personal problem in strictly intellectual terms and excludes all feeling and emotion from consciousness. For example, a patient, when talking of the severe abuse he experienced as a child, discusses his family's structure and conflicts, but expresses no emotion when mentioning his father's abusiveness.
17. *Interpersonal:* "That which takes place between persons" and/or that which characterizes "processes which arise as a result of the interaction of individuals" (Chaplin, 1975, pp. 267-268).
18. *Intrapsychic:* "Taking place within the personality or mind, such as intrapsychic conflicts which are expressions of the existence of two opposing motivations or impulses within the individual" (Chaplin, 1975, p. 269).
19. *Junior:* see also Unconscious. A synonym for the unconscious coined by Agnes Sanford to personify the rebellious, unruly part of herself. "For what I want to do I do not do, but what I hate I do" (Romans 7:15).
20. *Psychologically Unavailable:* A term used to describe an individual who is defensive, rigid, and resistant to the therapeutic process. Such individuals do not voluntarily seek professional psychological assistance. If they do involve themselves in psychotherapy, they generally terminate therapy prematurely.

21. *Repression (an ego defense):* "The forceful ejection from consciousness of impulses, memories, or experiences that are painful or shameful and generate a high level of anxiety. Repression, according to Freudian psychoanalysis, is a function of the ego" (Chaplin, 1975, p. 454) and "like all defense mechanisms, it is itself an unconscious process" (Walrond-Skinner, 1986, pp. 297-298). For example, most people repress their murderous rage at a parent who punishes them unfairly.

22. *Repression Barrier:* The conscious ego is defended from ongoing inevitable unconscious conflicts between the superego and the id (parent and child) by the repression barrier. It contains the defenses used to keep the individual unaware so he can attend to managing his daily affairs in the world. The repression barrier has affective and cognitive components.

23. *Self-Actualization:* "The innate capacity of human beings to grow and develop emotional and psychological maturity. The term is used by most humanistic therapists to describe the central motivating tendency in life" (Walrond-Skinner, 1986, p. 307).

24. *Somatization (an ego defense):* A process in which an individual expresses his psychic conflicts in physical manifestations. For example, an individual who is fearful of performing in a recital develops a severe headache that is so intense, he is unable to perform.

25. *Sublimation (an ego defense):* see also Haass. One of the five "higher level defenses." Sublimation means putting energy into areas other than those we cannot change. It involves disengaging from hopeless tasks and engaging in productive activities.

26. *Superego:* That part of the psychic apparatus which mediates between ego drives and social ideals, acting as a conscience that may be partly conscious and partly unconscious.

27. *Unconscious:* see also Junior. "The term is used both as a adjective and as a noun in psychoanalytical theory. Used adjectively, the term is a description applied to certain mental contents which are not currently within the individual's consciousness. These include both the contents of the preconscious and the system unconscious. Used as a noun, the term refers to the system unconscious, the region of the mind which remains unavailable to the individual, until it emerges into consciousness through certain products (dreams), processes (word associations, free association and parapraxes), or behaviors (symptoms) …. For psychoanalytic therapists, the root to understanding and treating psychological problems lies through the unconscious and symptoms viewed as conscious manifestations of unconscious conflicts" (Walrond-Skinner, 1986, pp. 372-373).

Key Word References
American Psychiatric Association. (1987). *Diagnostic and Statistical Manual of Mental Disorders (Third Edition – Revised)*. Washington, DC: American Psychiatric Association.

Campbell, R.J. (1981). *Psychiatric Dictionary – Fifth Edition*. New York & Oxford: Oxford University Press.

Chaplin, J.P. (1975). *Dictionary of Psychology – Revised Edition*. New York: Dell Publishing Co., Inc.

Drever, J. (19720. *A Dictionary of Psychology*. Baltimore, MD: Penguin Books.

Walrond-Skinner, S. (1986). *A Dictionary of Psychotherapy*. London & New York: Routledge & Kegan Paul.

Chapter 12

An Overview of a Spirit-Directed Therapy Session

Joseph Scerbo, S.A., Ph.D.
Mission San Juan Capistrano
P.O. Box 697
San Juan Capistrano, CA 92693

Practitioner

Joseph Scerbo, S.A., Ph.D. is a Franciscan Friar of the Atonement. His Ph.D. in Religion and Personality Sciences is from Graduate Theological Union, U.C. Berkeley, Berkeley, CA. He currently serves as Academic Dean and Faculty member at Trinity College of Graduate Studies, Anaheim, CA.

Journey of Integration

When I was first ordained, I prayed that my priesthood would not be limited between two candles. I did not know the full extent of that which I was asking. While the sacramental and liturgical dimension of my experience of priesthood continued to unfold, I felt my consciousness expanding to include the discovery of energizing life in its many forms.

Several years after my ordination to the priesthood, I felt drawn to explore the findings of psychology with what I was experiencing as a priest. I did not see at the time how my ordination prayer/request was to unfold. The following remarkable encounters served to shape my life, ministry, and experience of priesthood. The focus of my ministry has emerged as a result of the impact of these significant encounters in my life/unfoldment.

It was during the Fall of 1970 that I arrived in Berkeley to begin a doctoral program in what I perceived to be *bridge work* between the field of psychology and spirituality. During the first year of my work, I found myself interning as a group therapist in Tolman Hall's Psychology Clinic on the Berkeley Campus of the University of California. It was at the clinic that I met Claudio Naranjo, M.D.[1] His teaching threw the outlines of the chief feature of my own inner resistance to life/relationship into undeniable *high* relief. Part of the suffering that seems inevitable in such work was due, in my case, to the realization that my habitual functioning was organized around a central flaw or distortion of the truth that had much to do with wrong understanding. I am deeply grateful to him for enriching, inspiring, and challenging me. I learned a great deal about my *self* in that area of human experience, which the psychological school more traditionally defines as *resistance* to life/relationship.

Coinciding with this period of *apprenticeship* with Dr. Naranjo, I found myself further exploring *ways and means* of tilling the soil of my own experience. At *The Western Institute for Family and Group Therapy* in Watsonville, CA, I began supervised training in the principles and practices of Transactional Analysis[2] combined with Gestalt Therapy.[3] I am indebted to Dr. Robert and Mary Goulding[4] for the therapeutic skills I learned in *gathering the fragments* of my own experience and integrating these fragments more deeply into my life. My experience of both Mary and Bob Goulding plus Claudio Naranjo in the therapeutic setting was akin to watching an *artwork* unfold.

During the entire time I was working with Claudio Naranjo and Mary and Bob Goulding, I continued to experience my ministry as a priest taking on a variety of forms, ranging from teaching and directing retreats to preaching and administering the sacraments. I began to discover how psychological training could assist one's ministry. An added tool I found (in becoming aware of my own unique experience and in working through my resistance to emotional growth) was the imaging faculty. This tool was first introduced to me through the late Roberto Assagioli, M.D.[5] I am thankful for the personal contact I had with him in his home in Fiesole, Italy, in 1973. I felt his presence radiate energetic enthusiasm and delightful good humor. I am especially grateful to him for helping me to appreciate more fully the relationship of humor to health.

Throughout the remaining *seventies* I was exposed to groups of Christians who had learned to allow the energy within faith to overcome resistances to life/relationship and to bring about personality transformation. I perceived the healthy need for ongoing reconciliation with self, others, and God. As both priest and therapist, I saw reconciliation as a key to health and harmony, emotional and spiritual growth. A pertinent question that emerged for me within the reconciliation process was this: How does one come to the precise healing or learning that is potential in a personal hurt or loss so that the new strengths released for mutual upliftment enable one to combine vulnerability with confidence, sensitivity with strength, loving and compassion with effectiveness and integrity? From my experience as a priest, I found the biggest block to learning and growth was denial and repression of pain and the lack of self-acceptance. I began to see that psychotherapy and other humanistic growth techniques which could assist one in discovering what one genuinely feels beneath denial and self-judgment are not only compatible with Christian interiorization but could be extremely helpful. I concluded what a Carmelite contemplative and spiritual director so aptly described:

> The divinizing process which leads to transforming union, the ultimate stage of the Mystic Way, depends upon a healthy and harmonious indi-

viduation .... "Grace" does not destroy nature ... it perfects it, according to St. Thomas Aquinas (*Summa Theologiae*). Psychology can make an enormous contribution to the Christian mystical tradition by helping us to understand and foster the psychologically integrated man, who can thus be far more receptive to the workings of the divine in him than the unintegrated, disintegrated, or maladjusted man. This neither denies the reality of God's intervention nor overestimates the value of a psychology of Christian mysticism. It merely keeps things in proper perspective.[6]

In the late *seventies* I learned of The Association of Christian Therapists (ACT). At their biannual meetings, I discovered an exciting support system of men and women in the healing ministries who had academic and clinical preparation in the health care fields or who were actively involved in the Christian healing ministry. I became aware during the meetings that all the members of ACT were overwhelmingly convicted that healing through the power of Christ is valid for emotional and relational life.

During this same period of time I was led to meet a group of Christian psychologists, Dr. William Carr,[7] Dr. Douglas Schoeninger,[8] Sister Betty Igo, S.F.P.,[9] who were developing a Christ-oriented psychotherapy center. The Institute for Christian Healing had been in existence for three years when I became part of the staff. The cardinal value held by all those who worked at the Institute was the necessity for an utter and moment-by-moment dependence on the protection, inspiration, and leading of the Holy Spirit in the conduct of therapy. This meant that no fixed therapeutic strategy need be maintained. The foundation of the Institute rested upon 1) the individual prayer life of the staff, 2) the staff's own need for healing through prayer with one another, 3) the ongoing training in psychotherapy and human growth, and 4) the development of a close and loving community life together.

I spent three years working at the Institute for Christian Healing* in Narberth, PA as a staff therapist. Each week I saw sixteen clients individually for one-hour sessions. These clients came with a wide range of emotional and relational difficulties. All of them were *believing Christians* who desired to grow spiritually as well as emotionally. The ministry there was one of *inner healing* and acknowledging more fully the person that the Father has called us to be.

In my research I also came across the writings of Robert Campbell, S.J.

---

* The name was later changed to The Institute for Christian Counseling and Therapy. The Institute is now located at 1515 West Chester Pike, A-3, West Chester, PA 19382, 610-431-4730, email: DFLegacy@aol.com and James McPolin, S.J. and through them received deeper theological, pastoral insight into the practical content of the doctrine of the Scriptural "I Am." And my reading encounter with Howard Clinebell expanded and supported my own experience of human growth systems.

My struggle and integration of my priesthood with that of my personal and clinical experience continues to develop as my consciousness is challenged to grow by continuing to meet life in its various forms.

Methodology/Theology

In Spirit-Directed Therapy, as in most therapies, the client is brought into the place selected for therapy and is aided to relax and make the transition from small talk into his/her chosen area of therapeutic focus for that day. If a type of insightful prodding was given at the end of the preceding session, some attention is paid to the observation and/or questions the client might have before opening a new area of therapeutic endeavor.

After the area of intention is agreed upon and discussed, the therapist and client together open themselves to Jesus, the Master Therapist and Lord of the session, with a prayer similar to the following: "Lord, open those doors within me that you want open and take from me whatever is not for your glory. Fill me with your love and courage and help me face whatever truth you want to reveal this day. Close any doors of distraction and confusion that I am not ready to face and keep me from avoidance, postponement and denial of truth out of fear. Place me in the center of your perfect will."

Together the therapist and the client listen and relate the leadings they feel moved to bring into focus. They may be feelings, memories or ideas that arose during the prayer or they may be dreams, questions or concerns that the client intended to bring to the session in the preparation before arrival.

The modes of therapeutic endeavor are eclectic and vary from session to session, client to client. Whatever the modality is that is utilized in bringing one's experience into the light, the spiritual focus remains the same: the call of the Father, the reconciling love of Jesus Christ, and the power of the Holy Spirit to set one free. One's effort in this kind of therapy is to help the client to pass through the death-resurrection of Jesus. The client is invited to ask God's help in opening and closing areas of the heart. By doing this he/she shows a willingness to die to the *old* and take on new ways of thinking, feeling, and acting under the guidance of the Holy Spirit. Often what appears bound is released in the form of a new gift, a sense of aliveness not experienced before, and an expression of being that allows the *I am* to stand revealed in a new dimension. Whatever the modality, be it Transactional Analysis, Gestalt Therapy, Psychosynthesis, etc., sensitivity is given to the direction and leadings of the Holy Spirit working through that particular modality in the session.[10]

At the end of the session there is often a type of prayer asking Jesus to take any negative feelings ready to move into his redemptive act and replace these negative energies with transformed positive ones. "Christ himself carried our sins in his body to the cross, so that we might die to sin and live for righteousness. It is by his wounds that you have been healed" (I Pet. 2:24).

The Christian therapist often summarizes and gives some encouragement and/or possible direction for preparation for the next session. Prayer journaling, relaxation, and physical exercise are often encouraged. The case illustration following is an example of a session.

Context
The client in this case was seen at the Institute for Christian Healing, an out-patient psychotherapy center.

Goal
The client's initially stated goal was to deal with pain from a breakup in a very loving relationship.

Case Illustration
The individual who came to the author seeking help was a 35-year-old white male of Greek descent. When this person came to the first session, he was not at all in touch with his sadness or his anger. The pain of his loss was held inside since the breakup of his relationship. A whole year had elapsed before he had chosen to seek help.

In the successive sessions, the author learned that this man had a mother who tried to manipulate his father and his father possessed a quality of anger that was destructive (e.g., this person's father would break furniture when he was angry). One fear, which this client later discovered was his fear that *his* sadness would be like his mother's, i.e., very manipulative. Subconsciously, he also feared that his anger would be like his father's anger, i.e., very explosive and destructive. This first session was transcribed with the client's permission. It is an example of how prayer therapy unfolds.

First Session
Therapist (Joe): Hi, Tom, (A) I feel your pain already. A lot has been surfacing, hasn't it?

Client (Tom): (Gulp!) Yep. (Tom bites his lips. (B) Some tears begin to rise up to his cheeks and lodge themselves there. A smile appeared on his face to cover up the pain. With head drooped, Tom sighed.) I just keep on avoiding something. Yet I feel it's so close. (Tom looks at me.)

Joe: Yes, I know, Tom. Could we focus in now on the Lord in whatever way is best for you? Get in touch, first, with the rhythm of your breathing.

(C) Take some deep breaths. Allow yourself to experience your body. (Tom begins to close his eyes. He starts to breathe slowly.) Breathe out any tensions, anxiety, fears and let us ask the Holy Spirit to guide us into the truth. Continue with your breathing for a while. (Silence follows for about 60 seconds.) Now, if this seems right to you, Tom, could you repeat after me?

Tom: Okay.

Joe: Lord, open all those doors that will lead me to the truth and, Lord, close all those doors that will not lead me to the truth. Place me in the center of your perfect will. (D) (Tom repeats the prayer.) Okay. Now, Tom, can you imagine a large door on a heart and see yourself before that door? (E)

Tom: ... yes, I can see the door (pause) ... I am afraid to open it. I am turning away.

Joe: Okay. Now, Tom, can you allow yourself through the use of your imaging faculty to see Jesus enter into your sight and allow him to open the door with you?

Tom: I see ... I feel his presence in me opening the door. I am still afraid. I am still wanting to run. (F)

Joe: In the scripture we find the phrase, "Perfect love casts out fear" (I John 4:18). Can you repeat that, Tom?

Tom: Perfect love cast out fear ... perfect love cast out fear ... perfect love casts out fear. (Tom says this very slowly and very receptively.)

Joe: Can you return your attention, Tom, now to the door and allow the Spirit within you to bring up what needs to be looked at?

Tom: I see all these bats flying out ... it looks like a scene from one of Alfred Hitchcock's movies.

Joe: What is happening now? What are you experiencing?

Tom: Fear. I am afraid. I feel a pit in my stomach. I feel a little bit queasy. (G)

Joe: Can you, Tom, now image a cross? It is the cross of Jesus through which flows his redemptive love. (Pause) Can you image that?

Tom: Yes.

Joe: Okay. Now, can you see the word *fear* before you? If this helps, see the letters for fear appear F-E-A-R. Now can you see fear moving towards the cross?

Tom: I see the cross and I see dark clouds inside me being drawn into the light of the cross.

Joe: Good. Relax into where you are a little bit more. Now see the word *truth* coming back to you through the light of the cross.

Tom: I see light taking the form of fire (I) and this firelight is penetrating my being.

Joe: Good. Stay there a while and experience that. (A few minutes elapse.) Now let's return to what the *bats* might have to say to you. Can you

allow that image to return to you – the one that you saw before?
Tom: Okay. I can see them again. They are like mythological harpies that are harassing me ....
Joe: Okay. Now, in your imagination, switch roles (J) and allow the voices of the harpies to speak to you. You don't have to be afraid of them.
Tom: This is crazy ... okay ... (pause) – I know this is stupid, but I just feel the impact of their harassment saying, "You are wrong ... you are wrong ... you are wrong ... you are wrong ...."
Joe: What are you feeling, Tom?
Tom: I am afraid. I want to hide ... I have a feeling I'll be cut off from oxygen ... I can feel my chest get tight and my stomach feels like it fell in.
Joe: Was there ever a time, Tom, in your early life as a kid, where you had a similar feeling arise? Allow a scene to emerge from your past where this was so. (K)
Tom: Okay.
Joe: How old are you?
Tom: I am nine years old and I see myself with my father. My dad is working on the engine of his car. He is sweating and seems very tense and nervous. I am shinning a flashlight on the engine where my father is working and I drop the flashlight accidentally. Suddenly, dad jolts me with a scream, "What the hell is the matter with you? Don't you know how to do anything? What are you, *stupid*?" Wow ... I really feel that echo inside. It is like the word *stupid* is bouncing me all over the place. I don't feel anything. I freeze.
Joe: Stay with your breathing.
(Note: I perceived that Tom was re-experiencing this past picture frame and the corresponding emotional state of fear of his father's judgment. Fear caused him to choke off the expression of his out breath. I asked him to get back in touch with his full breathing pattern so that he could experience his experience.) Tom refocuses on his breathing.
Joe: (Pause) What are you feeling now?
Tom: I'm scared. I want to run. I want to cry ... oh, this is crazy, but I'm getting another image. It's a memory. I see myself flying through the air. My father and I had been wrestling on the floor and he threw me away from him in play and I loosened a tooth. I was scared then, too. I see that I am bleeding slightly and my dad comes over and with his strong hands on my shoulders says to me, "Thada boy. You didn't even cry." I felt as though I had achieved something.
(Note: Part of Tom's inability to cry and to experience the pain of his emotional loss originated with some early nonverbal parental injunctions that were evidenced in the past picture frames contained in his memory bank. Tom's interior hurts contained the memory of the judgment of his father. To win daddy's love, the early young Tom suppressed his tears, fear and anger.)

Joe: Okay, Tom, now I want to invite you back to face your father again. Allow yourself to get in touch with any unfinished business with him. In other words, what is it that you want to communicate to him? Image your father before you, Tom, and speak to your dad as if he were here now.

Tom: I am afraid of being yelled at again.

Joe: Can you give that over again, Tom, the word *fear*? Can you see fear going towards the cross? I am imaging the words FEAR OF JUDGMENT. Can you see those words move towards the cross?

Tom: Yes.

Joe: Now return your attention to your father and tell him what's so for you.

Tom: Daddy, I hurt ... you hurt me ....

Joe: Say that again.

Tom: Daddy, *you* hurt me!

Joe: Now exaggerate (L) that even more. Let your body move with your feelings. (A large pillow is next to Tom. I give it to him, encouraging him to use his arms to hit the pillow.)

Tom: Daddy, *you* hurt me (M) ... (he starts to pound the pillow with his fists) ... *you hurt* me ... *you hurt me*! ... I hate you ... (Tom continues to punch out the pillow.) I hate you!

(Note: Now Tom breaks down into deep sobbing. (N) In the same moment that I reached out to him, he reached out to me. I caught him in my arms. He continued to sob. I found myself stroking his head and gently rocking him back and forth.)

Joe: Just stay where you are, Tom. Give yourself permission to be. I am going to take on the role of your dad for a moment. (Pause) Son, I am sorry for yelling at you. I didn't mean to hurt you, honest. I didn't know what I was saying. Will you forgive me, son?

Tom: (Long pause) ……….. I forgive you, dad.

Joe: I am receiving an image, Tom, of you and your father. What I am seeing is the child within you and the child within your dad. Jesus has both of them by his hands and he is taking them out to play. Can you imagine that, Tom?

Tom: I can see the two of them playing marbles ... and now we are building a tree house together. Jesus is providing us with the material to build our house together.

Joe: Good. Now, when the house is finished, offer Jesus a seat and allow yourself to crawl up into his lap. Can you do this, Tom?

Tom: Yes.

Joe: Okay. Now allow yourself to feel the warmth of his love for you. How do you feel?

Tom: It feels good.

Joe: Would you be willing to change the word "it" to "I?"
Tom: Okay ... *I* feel good.
Joe: Now, once again, allow yourself to remain in Jesus' arms and receive whatever it is the Lord wants to give you.
(Note: At this point, a stillness came upon me with an inner prompting to reach out to Tom. Holding him in my arms, I began to hum to him using gibberish syllables. When it felt right, I shared with Tom what I was intuitively hearing underneath the sounding gibberish. (O) The words I received after each expression unfolded as the following.)

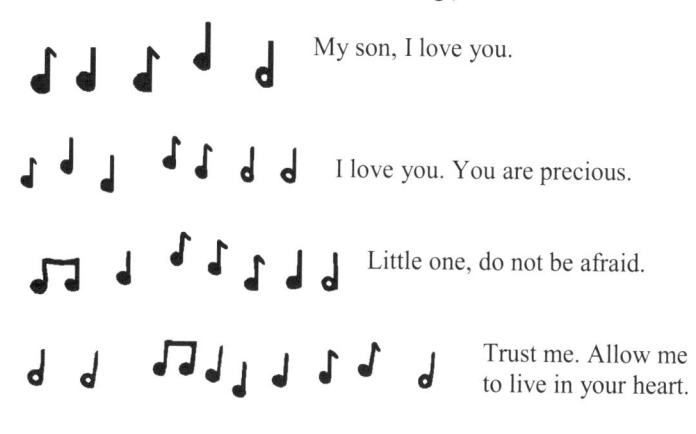

♪ ♩ ♪ ♩ ♩   My son, I love you.

♪ ♩ ♪ ♩ ♪ ♩ ♩   I love you. You are precious.

♫ ♩ ♪ ♪ ♪ ♩ ♩   Little one, do not be afraid.

♩ ♩ ♫ ♩ ♪ ♩ ♪ ♪ ♩   Trust me. Allow me to live in your heart.

♪ ♩ ♩ ♩ ♩ ♩ ♩ ♩ ♩   I love you. I am with you always.

(A moment of quiet followed. I continued to hold Tom until it was right to begin to end the session with a prayer of gratitude.) (P)

Lord, Jesus, we thank you and praise you for the time you have given us to be with each other. I thank you for the doors you opened for Tom today in this session, and I ask that the healing which you have begun be continued in the time, manner and intensity that is good for Tom. Thank you for freeing Tom from his fear of judgment and thank you for releasing the gift of tears within him. Guide him, Lord, throughout this day and throughout this evening. Continue to speak to him, Lord, at a place within his being that is beyond words. Allow him to be fed on the bread of your fidelity to him. Fill him with the peace of your holy name as he leaves here ... (Q) (Long pause) We'll see you next week, Tom.
Tom: Thanks, Joe.
Joe: Thank you, Tom.

Analysis of the Session (Note that the letters A, B, C, etc. below refer to specific places in the transcript indicated by the Letters A, B, C, etc.)

(A) It is well for the reader to know that the therapist had already spoken to Tom on the phone before he came into the office. He related something of his experiences. The inability to experience the pain of being separated from his loved one created for him more pain. It was this pain that became a factor in his own awareness that he needed help. The energy that he wanted to release as sadness and anger became bottled up and Tom became very depressed. Almost a whole year had passed in avoiding his pain, his anger and his sadness. The shock input of this rupture in relationship began to draw him into a much greater openness to knowing himself. The author saw this as drawing him more deeply into the call of the Father, the death-resurrection of Jesus and the power of the Holy Spirit to unbind him from his own fears and avoidance.

(B) Tom bites his lips to cover up the pain. Intense pain begins to emerge from the client. At the same time that the pain begins to surface, so does the negative conditioning within him stemming from his relationship with his father, which is later revealed in the session. At an early age, Tom learned to repress his experience of pain and perceived a reward with positive emotional stroking from his father. To experience pain and to communicate it to someone else, for Tom, would mean, subconsciously, to risk his father's disapproval, spoken or unspoken. So, as the pain from his loss started to emerge, so did some early emotional scenes with Father.

(C) By directing Tom to focus on his breathing, the therapist invites him to bypass his thoughts and allow his feelings to come up to the surface. The experience of doing nothing but attending to the contents of awareness may lead to a self-rewarding contact with reality, or to intense discomfort. If the therapist's view is correct, the technique of tabooing intellectual formulations may be seen as something like what the developer is to the photographic film: a means of bringing into light what otherwise might have remained invisible. The author thinks this is one thing that may be said of suppressive techniques in general. If one stays away from intellectualizations, one will sooner or later:
1. realize that one does not need them to gain self-knowledge; and
2. stumble upon the *holes* in one's personality: the areas of impotence, paralysis, inability to accept experience and discover the places that need the reconciling love of Jesus Christ and the power of the Holy Spirit to be set free.

(D) Oftentimes a short prayer at the beginning of each session helps to keep that spiritual focus that grounds this kind of therapy in the call of the Father, the reconciling love of Jesus Christ and the power of the Holy Spirit to set one free. If a client is open to prayer focus, the author usually begins this way. The author simply calls this an expression of *a prayer of the obedient heart*. In this prayer the whole session is placed under the Lordship of Jesus Christ and the guidance of the Holy Spirit.

(E) Much has been written on the use of imagery and metaphor in the therapeutic process. One individual who developed Desoille's "Guided Imagery" approach in therapeutic processes was Roberto Assagioli. In 1973, I had the opportunity of studying under Dr. Assagioli's direction in Fiesole, Italy. Imagery, he told us, serves to help the individual to contact the unconscious directly. The technique of imaging a heart over which there is a door to enter is one such example. In *Therapeutic Metaphors*[11] David Gordon exposes the role of metaphor in the therapeutic process: "Generally, a metaphor is defined as a way of speaking in which one thing is expressed in terms of another, whereby this bringing together throws new light on the character of what is being described" (p. 17).

(F) Tom's fear and anxiety are a damper signal anticipating the attack of the father. To ward himself off from expected harm, he developed defense mechanisms that prevented further hurt.

(G) The emotionally charged imagery of the *bats* manifests the negative aspects of those defenses. Dormant content within this image begins to emerge as the session unfolds. There are many different ways one can react to what one fears. These are some. This man chose a mixture of 2 and 3.

1. Attack

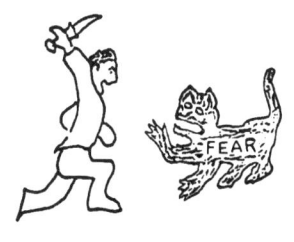

2. Flee

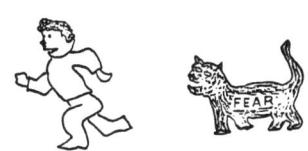

3. Avoid

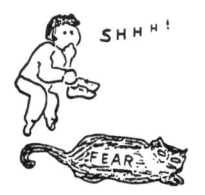

4. Neglect

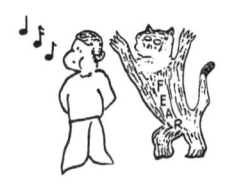

5. Succumb

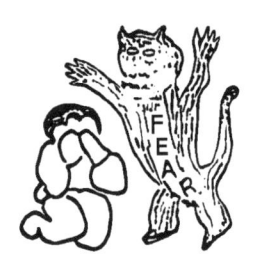

(H) The *cross* is one symbol of healing and transformation. As one is drawn into the death-resurrection of Jesus, the inner resistances, indolence, bitter resentment, pride, vanity, melancholy, avarice, fear, gluttony and punitiveness lose their grip and a newness of life and love emerges in whatever the Father calls one to be. Through the technique of imaging the *cross* the author finds that clients are given the chance to say *yes* internally to the redemptive act of Jesus Christ on the cross.

(I) Different symbols will spontaneously emerge within the consciousness of a client within a session. Tom began to image fire. One Christian interpretation of *fire* is this: fire is a symbol that St. Luke uses to tell us about the sign the Holy Spirit chose to make known his presence on Pentecost. God's presence was compared to *tongues as of fire* (Acts 2:3). The author is not equating this client's experience of fire with Luke's experience. The author merely wants to illustrate our need of symbols to embrace our healing and our religious experience.

(J) Dramatization of subselves can often serve to help the client to become aware of what he/she is avoiding in life, what he/she is failing to acknowledge, allow or express, and yet is part of himself/herself. In helping clients to express the precise aspects of themselves that they are suppressing, one is helping them to know themselves, to take responsibility for what *is* and thus to invite wholeness into their experience. As seen in this dramatization of this client's fear of judgment, implicit content is made explicit.

(K) Oftentimes a truth process seems to unfold that the author can describe as follows: For clients dealing with major emotions like fear, depression, guilt, anger, etc., the Christian therapist invites the client to:

1. *Experience* that emotion and discover where that particular emotion is experienced in the *body*;
2. Initiate an inquiry by asking the client if there was a time in the past when he/she experienced almost the same feeling;
3. Close his/her eyes and to allow a scene to emerge when he/she felt a similar feeling *back then* and to observe, a) "How old are you and b) what is happening in the scene, describing the position of your body in relation to others in that scene;"
4. Express *attitudes* experienced about himself/herself, others, God, as a result of that historic early experience;
5. Enumerate decisions made as a result of those attitudes;
6. Invite the Risen Jesus into the picture frame or memory and follow the client's experience moment by moment.

(L) This is a method, the purpose of which is to intensify the client's awareness of a given action or statement, and may be seen as a step beyond the Christian therapist's action of simply mirroring or reflecting. Exaggeration or repetition may have a dramatic effect in that the person brings himself/herself to see more and more wholeheartedly something that was minimized or not weighed fully, or was covered up under a mask. When a person is asked to exaggerate and does this a number of times, something new may be discovered or perhaps something that is not completely new, but that lay in the person's original behavior, like an invisible seed, so that only exaggeration could make it obvious.

(M) The Christian therapist invites the client to confront dad. In effect, this is *doing what is avoided*. By making this protest, the client accepts the *fact* that the rejection from his father did actually occur and realizes that all efforts to deny the fact are a waste of energy. One is bound to the past if the memory and feelings associated with it are repressed. While repression of memory is a psychological process, suppression of feelings is accomplished by deadening a part of the body or reducing its motility so that feeling is diminished. It was observed in the case illustration that the body structure of this person showed a barrel chest and that the structure of his chest indicated a *holding in* of feeling, especially anger and sadness. Even as the client was asked to breathe slowly, his *out breath* appeared shallow and interrupted, indicating an inability to express what feelings were inside him.

(N) Many people adopt roles, wear masks, and *play games*, because they do not believe their genuine self is acceptable. This man believed that his tears were not acceptable. Consequently, he put on a smiling mask to be lovable and adopted a façade of manliness. Most roles develop subtly in response to unspoken demands and pressures from significant others. *Breaking down* for this man amounts to a *breaking through*, allowing the love of Jesus to fill a deep, unmet need from this person's father.

(O) Gibberish is one of the few actions that cannot be programmed or rehearsed. Willingness to *speak* gibberish, used either by the client or Christian therapist or both, may be seen as a willingness to say the unknown, the unthought. Gibberish obediently molds itself to our inner reality, as an artwork. Putting words into gibberish often leads to expanded awareness. Tom's energy that was bound by the fear of his father's judgments was released with acceptance of the unacceptable parts within him, the right to cry and express fear. He was moved in the session towards an experience of forgiveness with his father and with himself. The tongue-speaking at the end of the session expressing the reconciling and affirming love of God for Tom could be seen to be what William Samarin calls "a linguistic symbol of the sacred ... a precious possession, a divine gift" Cf. *Tongues of Men and Angels*[12] (Samarin, 1972), p. 231; cf. *The Psychology of Speaking in Tongues* [13] (Kildahl, 1972), Chapter Two, "How Tongue Speakers Describe What They Do (Eighteen Questions Answered)" and Chapter Seven, "Psychological Factors in the Glossolalia Experience, pp. 57-65.

(P) The uniqueness of this kind of therapy as compared to secular therapy is the faith-belief in God's *I am* and a moment-by-moment dependence on the Holy Spirit which is given to:

1. unite us with Jesus Christ in his death, burial, and resurrection (Rom. 6:1-11, Col. 2:12);
2. to effect new birth, new creating, newness of life (Jn. 3:5; Titus 3:5);
3. to offer, give, and assure us of the forgiveness of sins in both cleansing and life-giving aspects (Acts 2:38);
4. to enable our continual repentance and daily reception of forgiveness, and our growing in grace;
5. to create unity and equality in Christ (I Cor. 12:13; Gal. 3:27-28);
6. to make us participants in the new age initiated by the saving act of God in Jesus Christ (Jn. 3:5); and
7. to place us into the Body of Christ where the benefits of the Holy Spirit are shared within a visible community of faith (Acts 2:38; I Cor. 12:13).

(Q) Infilling prayer is very important at the end of a session. The Christian therapist can pray with the client that Jesus replace any of the hurts or deceits with his love and peace. Unless the person's real needs are met, the false solutions and unhappiness will continue to rob that person of his peace.

Summary and Discussion

In this case illustration some of the more important tasks of the Christian therapeutic endeavor were set forth in:

- helping the client to recognize and remove blocks to the truth of what the Father has called him/her to be and
- helping the client to explore the areas of forgiveness and the benefits forgiveness has in his or her life.

A verbatim of a session in Spirit-Directed Therapy was presented with an analysis of what unfolded in that session.

Two themes from the session invite comment. There are two dimensions of growth within the client's life. One is the personal dimension. The other is the transpersonal dimension. They are distinct but not separate.

In the last decade, a growing number of psychologists have said that both dimensions are essential to full human growth, and they have begun to explore the relation between them. Andra Angyal, for example, discusses not only the individual's need to achieve autonomy, but also his/her need for the experience of *homonomy*, or union with a greater whole.[14]

In a similar way, Roberto Assagioli has recognized and developed two inter-related aspects of psychosynthesis: personal psychosynthesis, which aims at fostering the development of a well-integrated, effective personality, and spiritual psychosynthesis, which leads to realizing one's higher nature.[15]

Abraham Maslow, who introduced the term *transpersonal*, arrived through his observations, at parallel conclusions. In his later work, Maslow recognized three groups of people whom he called, respectively: self-actualizers, transcenders, and transcending self-actualizers. Self-actualizers, Maslow found, are "essentially practical, realistic, mundane, capable and secular people," pragmatically concerned with "growth toward self-actualization and freedom from basic deficiency needs." Such people live in the world, coming to fulfillment in it. They master it, lead it, and use it for good purposes.[16]

Transcenders, as understood by Maslow, are seen as non-self-actualizers, that is, people who have important transcendent experiences and a strong contact with the spiritual dimension, but whose personalities are often underdeveloped. When compared to the transcenders in this concept, the self-actualizers "tend to be 'doers' rather than mediators or contemplators, effective and pragmatic rather than aesthetic, reality testing and cognitive rather than emotional and experiencing.[17]

Maslow found it necessary to differentiate between two kinds of self-actualizing people: Those who had little or no experience of transcendence but a healthy functioning ego, and those in whom transcendent experiencing was important and even central and have been able to relate these experiences in a healthy way through the functioning ego. These latter he called transcending self-actualizers.

Transcending self-actualizers, in addition to being well integrated, healthy and effective, possess a sense for the *sacred*. They value and are more easily aware of truth, beauty, God, goodness, and unity.[18]

For a Christian therapist as well as a client to express in a healthy manner the rhythm of Spirit-Directed Therapy, it is important for both to continually attempt to integrate experience through their functioning ego, as described of a transcending self actualizer.

Further, in the light of Christian revelation, Christians readily use the words *reconciliation* and *healing*. The author sees the living realities expressed by these words as a call to a moment-to-moment walk in the Spirit. The starting point of this life-long growth is God's love and goodness which is found in each person's call to be. For St. John, this starting point is found in the mystery, "In the beginning was the Word; the Word was in God's presence, and the Word was God" (Jn. 1:1, NAB). And, also, in the passage, "Through him all things came into being, and apart from him nothing came to be" (Jn 1:3, NAB). All growth arises out of the Father's love, who so loved the world to the point of giving it his only Son. In Jn. 3:3 (NAB) Jesus says, "I solemnly assure you, no one can see the reign of God unless he is begotten from above." To the Spirit-Directed therapist, this instruction implies the ongoing reconciliation and healing which is the basis for Spirit-Directed Therapy.

To sum up, then, a Christian is a pilgrim on the journey following Jesus into a *yes*, that is a fuller expression of one's authentic *I am*. This expression of the *I am* eventually comes to rest in the Triune unlimited *I Am* the more that the person experiences reconciliation and healing. This is the goal of Christ-centered, Spirit-Directed Therapy.

Footnotes

1. Claudio Naranjo is a very intriguing figure in the field of the Psychology of Religion. He is a Chilean-born psychiatrist and author of several books and monographs on psychology and meditation. *The Psychology of Meditation, The One Quest*, and *The Healing Journey* are samples of his contributions to the field of psychology and religion. As a direct disciple of Frederick ("Fritz") Perls, M.D., Claudio Naranjo has studied Gestalt Therapy, used it in his work, and made original contributions in this field.
2. An overview of this contemporary counseling and therapy model is taken from Gerald Corey, (1977). *Theory and Practice of Counseling and Psychotherapy*. Belmont, CA: Wordsworth Publishing Co., p. 72.

Transactional Analysis (TA) is an interactional psychotherapy that can be used in individual therapy but that is particularly apart from most other therapies in that it is both contractual and decisional. It involves a contract, developed by the client, that clearly states the goals and direction of the therapy process. It also focuses on early decisions that each person makes, and it stresses the capacity of the person to make new decisions and alter the course of his or her life.

The contractual nature of the psychotherapeutic process tends to equalize the power of the therapist and the client. It is the client's responsibility to decide what he or she will change. To make the changes a reality, the client changes behavior in an active manner. During the course of therapy, the client evaluates the direction of his or her life, comes to understand some very early decisions that he or she made, and realizes that he or she can now redecide and initiate a new direction in life. In essence, then, TA assumes that people can learn to trust themselves, think and decide for themselves, and express their feelings.
3. Ibid., p. 95.

Developed by Frederick Perls, Gestalt Therapy is a form of existential therapy based on the premise that individuals must find their own ways in life and accept personal responsibility if they hope to achieve maturity. As it works mainly on the principle of awareness, the Gestalt approach focuses attention on the *what* and *how* of behavior and experience in the here-and-now by integrating the fragmented and unknown parts of personality.

4. Mary Goulding, M.S.W., is a clinical social worker and Co-Director of The Western Institute for Group and Family Therapy. In the author's perception, Mary brings to her clinical work, her teaching, and her writing a keen theoretical mind, therapeutic skills that cut through superfluity and a gift for eye-widening confrontations that awaken rather than stun. Robert Goulding, M.D., is Co-Director with his wife, Mary, of The Western Institute for Group and Family Therapy. He is past President (1976-1978) of the American Academy of Psychotherapists, a fellow of both the American Group Psychotherapy Association and the American Psychiatric Association. Among his teachers were Eric Berne and Fritz Perls. Bob and Mary are both teaching members of the International Transactional Analysis Association.

In the author's perception, Bob blends an ability to nurture with a good sense of humor and makes changes in the here-and-now a safe adventure.

Bob and Mary have written, *The Power is in the Patient, a TA/Gestalt Approach to Therapy,* (1978). San Francisco: TA Press, and *Changing Lives Through Redecision Therapy.* (1979). New York: Brunner/Mazel.

5. Roberto Assagioli, who was born in Venice in 1888, is a significant figure of modern psychology in the line that runs from Freud through Jung and Maslow. Himself a colleague of all these men, Assagioli was among the pioneers of Freudianism in Italy, though he pointed out that Freud had largely neglected the higher reaches of human nature. Over the years, Assagioli developed a comprehensive psychology known as Psychosynthesis. Psychosynthesis is a psychotherapeutic approach and philosophy of education that seeks to integrate body, mind, and feelings with openness to the transpersonal dimensions of conscious experience.

6. William McNamara, O.C.D., (1978). "Psychology and the Christian mystical tradition," *Transpersonal Psychologies*, ed. Charles Tart, New York: Harper & Row, p. 391.

7. William L. Carr received his doctorate in Education from the University of Pennsylvania in 1971. In 1976 Dr. Carr founded The Institute for Christian Healing, Narberth, PA.

8. Before becoming Vice-President of The Institute for Christian Healing, Douglas W. Schoeninger, Ph.D., served as Family therapist for the Department of Family Psychiatry at Eastern Pennsylvania Psychiatric Institute. Doug's degree in Clinical Psychology is from the University of Wisconsin.

9. Sister Betty Igo, S.F.P., M.S., is a Franciscan Sister of the Poor, and for years has been involved in prayer counseling and teaching in the field of inner healing. Sister Betty conducts beginning and advanced training for ministers of healing in California and throughout the United States. She holds an M.S. in Guidance from Xavier University in Ohio.

10. Other modalities abound. One may, for example, attempt to set up new environmental learning situations by some sort of group therapy, open once again to the guidance of the Holy Spirit and the healing power of the Risen Lord Jesus. One may use behavior modification by observing the ways in which a mother, for example, reinforces a child's avoidance behavior and may work within to change these. One may see a mother individually to help her change her perception of mothering, support her in developing her self or involve her in sensitivity training. One can work with the father in exploring his frequent illnesses or in helping him to find more job satisfaction. One may select the modality of couple therapy to assist parents in dealing with their sexual problems and developing a more satisfactory marriage. And one may use family therapy to increase communication, clarify the parents' interactions with the child and find ways of modifying the influence of *significant others* in the child's life.

11. Gordon, D. (1978). *Therapeutic Metaphors: Healing Others Through the Looking Glass.* Cupertino, CA: Meta Publications.

12. Samarin, W. (1972). *Tongues of Men and Angels* New York: Macmillan Co., p. 231.

13. Kildahl, J.P. (1972). *The Psychology of Speaking in Tongues*. New York: Harper and Row.
14. Angyal, A. (1965). *Neurosis and Treatment: A Holistic Theory*. New York: Viking Press
15. Assagioli, R. (1993). *Psychosynthesis: A Manual of Principles and Techniques*. New York: Penguin USA.
16. Firman, J. and Vargui, J. (1977). "Dimensions of Growth," *Synthesis* 3.
17. Maslow, A. (1971). "Theory Z," *The Farther Reaches of Human Nature*. New York: Viking Press, pp. 280ff.
18. ibid.

Chapter 13

Grandfather's Fear*

Douglas W. Schoeninger, Ph.D.
1515 West Chester Pike, #A-3
West Chester, PA 19382

Practitioner
Douglas W. Schoeninger, Ph.D., Clinical Psychology, University of Wisconsin, 1965. Private practice of psychotherapy.

Training
Client Centered Therapy with Carl Rogers, Ph.D.; Contextual Family Therapy with Ivan Nagy, M.D. (see Boszormenyi-Nagy in references) and Barbara Krasner, Ph.D. Also trained in applied kinesiology and neuro-emotional techniques with Scott Walker, D.C. and Theresa Dale Ph.D, N.D. and in Healing the Family Tree through collaborations with Kenneth McAll, M.D.

Journey of Integration
I began integrating healing prayer with psychotherapy in 1974, learning first of healing prayer during my initial contacts with charismatic renewal at Narberth Presbyterian Church in Narberth, PA, where I became a member in 1973. My first experience of healing prayer occurred at a healing service where I witnessed the *laying on of hands* during prayers for individuals and experienced these prayers for myself, as I sought healing for depression. My first brief relief from a very debilitating depressed mood occurred after being prayed with during a healing service. In 1973 I met a psychologist interning at my place of employment (Eastern Pennsylvania Psychiatric Institute) who was a Christian and was also interested in these matters. My discussions with him eventually led, in 1975, to learning of the formation of The Association of Christian Therapists and about healing prayer workshops being given by Ruth Carter Stapleton. My first introduction to healing of memories prayer was through attending a workshop given by Ruth Carter Stapleton on Long Island. I was thrilled by the possibilities I could imagine for integrating healing prayer into psychotherapy. Attending this workshop then led to discussions about healing prayer with the ministers of my church and with other Christian therapists, and to the beginnings of trying inner healing and healing of memories prayers in psychotherapy sessions with Christian clients at

---

* First published in *The Journal of Christian Healing*, Volume 20, Number 3&4, Fall/Winter, 1998, pp. 77-85.

Eastern Pennsylvania Psychiatric Institute in the Family Psychiatry Department where I was employed. Later I joined the newly founded (1976) Institute for Christian Healing (ICH) in Narberth, PA, an organization founded for the purpose of integrating healing prayer and Christian spirituality with psychotherapy, was the perfect place to practice these newly found fledgling skills.

Gradually my training in Contextual Family Therapy, an intergenerational family model, began to integrate with inner healing and healing of memories prayer. On the one hand inner healing prayers would reveal, through the client's inner imagery and my inner imagery, root generational dynamics of the persons being prayed with. On the other hand, Contextual Family Therapy explorations would lead clients and myself into discovering and imagining the lives of the client's parents, grandparents and great grandparents, etc., preparing the ground for compassion and forgiveness for ancestors.

Through my work at the Institute for Christian Healing (later known as the Institute for Christian Counseling and Therapy), discussions with other staff members and then through membership in the Association of Christian Therapists, the development of this integration has continued.

Context

The context of this illustration is an outpatient psychotherapy practice, The Institute for Christian Counseling and Therapy (formerly The Institute for Christian Healing). The client, a female age 30, was referred to me by persons in healing ministry, acquainted with our practice, who had developed a trust and referral relationship with us. The client contracted for psychotherapy sessions on an every other week basis due to financial constraints.

Goal

The client's initially stated goal for therapy was to overcome fear and passivity, to learn to deal with her own anger and to set boundaries in relationships with her husband and her parents.

Theory/Theology

The vulnerabilities and dependencies of childhood leave no doubt that each generation is highly subject to its caretakers' provisions and presence, deprivations and absence. Clinical observation, as well as ordinary experience of parents with their children, reveal that parents' own rearing shapes to a marked degree their offerings. The stream of generation to generation influence therefore bears the marks of all that has been healed and all that remains broken and distorted as each generation creatively reforms or repetitiously copies its progenitors' ways.

Thus within persons and between persons, the unfinished business of one's ancestors, the disquieted relationships with self, God and others, call out for redemptive attention. This pull of unfinished business one may experience as intransigent (stuck, unchanging) emotion, fear, anxiety, grief, despair, anger, bouts of rage, or as repetitive patterns of action, such as compulsions and rigid patterns of relating, persistent distrust, defensiveness or blame. Ancestors' unsettled relations with God, self, others and the natural world in some sense indwell present generations and work between living persons with real though hidden force, pulling persons repeatedly into their field of influence.

The persistence of binding ancestral influences has been explained in various ways. Four possible dynamics or means of influence are (1) curses, (2) loyalties, (3) memories, and (4) the pressuring of the living by the departed who are not at rest.

(1) Some have pointed to the curse effects of the sins of ancestors to the third and fourth generations (Prince, 1990) as disclosed in Exodus 20:5: "For I, Yahweh your God am a jealous God and I punish a parent's fault in the children, the grandchildren, and the great grandchildren among those who hate me; ..." (NJB). Prince (1990) sees the curse effects of ancestors' sins as manifesting both in tendencies to be caught up in similar sinful patterns and in failures to thrive in life.

(2) Others (Nagy & Spark, 1973; Nagy & Krasner, 1986) point to ancestral pain and patterns mediated by loyalty, commitment of children to their parents and through parents to grandparents and more distant ancestors. Each generation invests in the lives of their forebears by helping to bear their burdens and by continuing their ways. There is a tendency to repeat ancestral patterns through unexamined loyalty to ancestors' ways of thinking, believing, behaving and relating.

(3) Yet a third means of influence may be the inheritance of parental and ancestral memories through inborn tendencies to react to situations and relationships as if one had lived one's ancestors' experiences. The means by which the memories of past generations may actively shape the present generation's consciousness have been examined in depth by Sheldrake (1988).

(4) Fourthly, McAll (1982, Smith, 1992, 1996; Hampsch, 1986; Linn, Linn & Fabricant, 1985) sees, in addition to the above influences, that living family members may be pressured by deceased ancestors who are seeking attention or intercession for their captive, troubled condition by, in some sense, visiting the living with their unquiet state.

From my point of view, these four dynamics or means of generational influence represent facets of a whole and different gates of entry into a healing process. Each dynamic calls for specific healing strategies.

Methodology

The healing methodology combined Contextual Therapy, addressing old injuries and current transactions within a framework of relational justice, with inner healing prayer, including healing of inherited ancestral memories which are imbedded in, and condition responses to, personal history. The sessions consisted of verbal explorations. The client responded to my questions and posing of options. These included options offered to stimulate her imagination for healing and justice-creating responses in relationships, and intrapsychic options, alternative ways she could respond to herself, parts of herself, and inner painful experiences in her interior imagination. Role playing relational options and dramatizing intrapsychic exchanges and options, for example, between her adult self and teenage self, were used to help the client translate concepts into action and then to bring to awareness additional fears and loyalty obligations that needed reworking for her to be free. Time was spent at the end of sessions teaching inner healing prayer and healing of memories imagery.

Given this client's active prayer life, she preferred being trained in prayer methods during the sessions and beginning the prayers during the sessions, then continuing healing prayers on her own time especially during Mass or when sitting before the Blessed Sacrament. Healing prayer methodologies included using active imagination, imagining the situations in which the wounds occurred, getting in touch with the wounding events by replaying them using all of the senses or by picturing them and feeling them for the first time, as in ancestral events, and inviting Jesus into those images to heal the wounds remembered and imagined.

Case Illustration

Client's Significant History

This client came to me bothered by persistent intense fears. Some of her fear she traced to childhood and intense exchanges with her father wherein he would suddenly and fiercely rage at her for *no apparent reason*. These rages instilled in her an almost constant fear of doing something wrong and of displeasing others. She said, "I blindly do what people want and usually apologize whether I've done anything or not." Investigation of her family tree (see Figure One) through her conversations with her father and other relatives revealed that her grandfather (her father's father) had entered the United States alone, as an illegal alien, and had spent some years surviving on the streets, hiding from authorities and in almost constant vigilance for fear of being caught. When my client learned this, she recognized the similarity of her fears to those she imagined her deceased grandfather had experienced and realized that her father's rages (which descended from Grandfather's fears) had the consequence of instilling these fears in her.

Figure 1: "K" Family

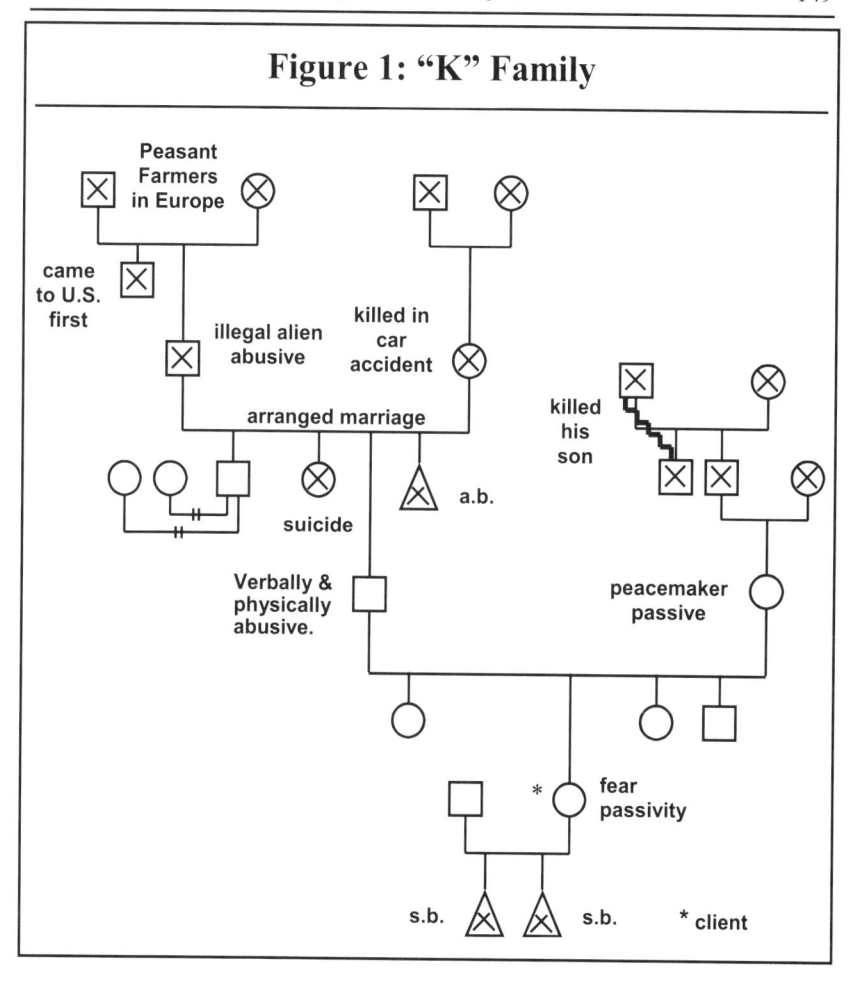

Figure showing genogram of the K Family with the following annotations:
- Peasant Farmers in Europe
- came to U.S. first
- illegal alien abusive
- arranged marriage
- killed in car accident
- suicide
- a.b.
- Verbally & physically abusive.
- killed his son
- peacemaker passive
- fear passivity
- s.b.
- s.b.
- * client

Healing, Interventions and Processes: Beginning/Getting Started

The initial session included the exploration of the client's complaint, her hopes for treatment, family history, and genealogy, especially regarding the generation to generation development of the issues with which she was struggling, and discussion of religious faith practice and experience. This initial exploration revealed her longstanding regular prayer life within Roman Catholic traditions. She regularly attended Mass and received Eucharist. She spent specific time daily praying upwards to one half hour, interceding for family and friends and petitioning regarding her own wounds and stuck places. She regularly engaged the Sacrament of Reconciliation. In spite of her intense and disciplined prayer life and moments of knowing and sensing

God's presence and love, she felt inwardly cut off from God and herself. She found herself in bondage to fear, paralyzed to act on her own behalf, always feeling guilty for negative relational outcomes, and pervasively apologetic.

This client made it known that she was seeking a psychotherapy centered in Christian faith and drawing on the power of prayer. She was open to and desired beginning our sessions with prayer and was responsive to my suggestions that we begin each session calling on the Holy Spirit to guide us, committing all that we did to the Lordship of Jesus and binding the powers of darkness. Thus, each session began with these prayers, prayed spontaneously in a dialogic, back and forth, manner between us.

In addition, I shared with this client a prayer for the binding of evil which she could use daily or when she experienced the need, for example praying silently when she feared impending violence with someone in the family.

When the client appeared for her third session two weeks later, she proceeded to unfold for me the content of her prayers and experiences while sitting before the Blessed Sacrament (an important part of her prayer practice) at her local parish church. She had confessed to Jesus her grandfather's sins, apologized on behalf of her grandfather, and voiced her grandfather's struggles as a young man. As she did this she received a very strong inner awareness of her grandfather's fears. She then spoke these fears to Jesus, bound Satan from them in the name of Jesus, and asked the Lord to heal her grandfather's wounds. Later she silently voiced these confessions and healing prayers during a parish Mass and received the Body and Blood of Jesus for the remission of his sins and the healing of his wounds. As she sat quietly after receiving the elements, my client prayed further that her father would now be released from fears and that he, also, would receive the benefits of this healing. Then she sat and inwardly envisioned Jesus. She saw in her mind's eye her grandfather made whole and joyful in Jesus' presence and then proceed on with Jesus into a bright light.

Following these prayer experiences, my client reported a significant lessening of fear and a remarkable change in her father, whom she now had the courage to address face to face. When she sat with her father and boldly told him how she had experienced his rages as a child, her father listened without defending. His receptivity was an entirely new behavior.

During the latter part of session three my client reported experiencing an urgency to pray for her miscarried babies. While she had spiritually cared for two stillbirths, she had previously not acknowledged other miscarriages. She imagined up to 15 and wanted to pray for them. In this case she preferred to pray in the session with my guidance. In her prayer imagery Jesus brought the babies to her. She named each child, held each, expressed her love to each and committed each to Jesus who then baptized each baby and handed each child into the arms of Mary. At the end of these prayers my client felt considerable relief, an inward lightening as if burdens had been lifted.

Midcourse Psychotherapy Process

In this case, generational healing prayers preceded other therapy and healing work. These prayers seemed to release spiritual and emotional burdens of fear and grief, and free energy and hope for surfacing and facing other issues. Subsequently her times of prayer between sessions seemed to facilitate a progressive awareness of wounds needing healing and attitudes requiring change. During each session she would express the contents of her prayer experiences between sessions.

Sessions 4 - 8

Focus on self hatred led to memories of sexual abuse during adolescence, and to release of long dissociated pain through tears as she prayed before the Blessed Sacrament. These therapy sessions then included follow-up to her prayer experiences before the Blessed Sacrament. Lengthy healing of memories prayers were engaged wherein Jesus was visualized entering the moments of abuse, removing her from the scene, restoring her body, cleansing her sexuality, clothing her in white.

A freedom to feel and to fully express emotions and felt experiences to Jesus began to increase. "In writing I told Jesus everything I felt. Then, in my imagination, he held me."

Sessions 9 - 13

The focus shifted to reworking relationships with her father and her husband. We discussed options for taking care of herself, for asserting boundaries, and making claims while considering others.
She reported:
"My father lit into me. I shot back at him .... In my prayer I saw the Lord cleansing the temple ...."
"... I used to try to calm my husband by trying to be perfect. That would infuriate him. Now I express anger back at him and we are beginning to talk it out."
"My sister, mother and husband are beginning to pray together weekly."

Follow-up and Conclusion

This session, number 14, was scheduled about a month after the previous session and turned out to be our final meeting. It consisted of a reporting of her experiences during the previous month and a crediting on my part of her faithful (and successful) pursuit of healing.
She reported:

- My father joined our family prayer group.
- Father dreamed that his father came to him saying, "I'm sorry."
- I completed a 33 day consecration to the Blessed Mother. I asked for the root of *reactive retaliation* to be taken. I felt this deep energy pulled out of me and a joy welling up in its place.
- I've stopped fixing my husband's pain.

Discussion

From the illustration given and the healing described the reader may already see how the four dynamics (curses and blessings, ancestral memories, generational loyalties, and prayer for the departed) may be combined. This case included all four dynamics. The curse of fear was broken through apologies made for the grandfather's many illegal and violent actions. The power of fear was revoked through receiving the Blood of Jesus for cleansing the effects of sin. One can see that the conscious and deliberate engagement of the resources offered in the consecrated bread and wine is a powerful way of receiving the exchange of life for death articulated so precisely by Prince in his work on curses and blessings (1990).

In addition this client actively pursued the reworking of loyalties by investigating the roots of her fears in her father's and grandfather's wounds and life struggles. Crediting their brokenness and then praying for their healing (a new way of honoring their lives) she gained the courage to *honor* her father by directly addressing him with her experience of his rage. Loyalty through silence and fear was gradually replaced by loyalty through claiming just consideration for all family members.

Healing grandfather's memories, which seemed imbedded in her own fears naturally evolved as she considered her father's and grandfather's lives while sitting before the Blessed Sacrament. She found herself imagining Jesus walking with her grandfather through the terrible isolation and terror of his separation from his family and his hidden illegal years. In this she *observed* and absorbed the power of Jesus' love healing her grandfather's terrible alienation.

Finally in her prayers for her grandfather during the Eucharistic liturgy, she saw him in the presence of Jesus, made whole and transported on in his journey with God into the light.

In this case, tending each dynamic, curses, loyalties, memories and release of the departed into Jesus' care seemed to deepen and strengthen the healing received. Each of the four dynamics of generational influence and healing presented here plays a powerful role in family life. The particular dynamics emphasized in healing will vary, however, family to family. Some of this variation has to do with the framework that is comfortable and workable for the family. For example, persons who do not believe in praying for the dead will not directly engage that dimension. However, they may be comfortable confessing their ancestors' sins and injuries in the context of breaking curses and healing memories.

In each case we seek the leading of the Holy Spirit in guiding our attention to these four dynamics. Whichever is emphasized, most often all four seem to play a part. Curses will be broken in the context of healing memories. Loyalties are implicitly reworked as ancestors' wounds are brought to light and their lives and struggles are reconsidered during preparation of prayers for the departed. Specific ancestral memories come to light for healing as roots of disobedience are exposed in the process of searching for the sources of a curse. Prayers for the departed proceed naturally from prayers for healing inherited wounds. Tending each dynamic adds a critical undergirding strength to the whole healing process.

References
Boszormenyi-Nagy, I., and Krasner, B. R. (1986). *Between Give and Take. A Clinical Guide to Contextual Therapy.* New York: Brunner/Mazel.

Boszormenyi-Nagy, I., and Spark, G.M. (1973). *Invisible Loyalties: Reciprocity in Intergenerational Family Therapy.* New York: Harper and Row.

Epstein, A.W. (1982). "Mental phenomena across generations: The holocaust," *Journal of the American Academy of Psychoanalysis. 10, 565-570.*

Fiore, E. (1987). *The Unquiet Dead.* New York: Ballantine Books.

Hampsch, J.H. (1986). *Healing Your Family Tree.* Everett, WA: Performance Press.

Linn, M., Linn, D. and Fabricant S. (1985). *Healing the Greatest Hurt.* Mahwah, NJ: Paulist Press.

McAll, K. (1992) *Conference on Healing the Family Tree.* West Chester, PA: Institute for Christian Counseling and Therapy (ICCT), set of ten audio tapes including prayers for departed ancestors (for a complete list of audio and video offerings on Generational Healing and other topics of Christian Healing from ICCT contact: Robin Caccese, 137 Proudfoot Drive, Birdsboro, PA 19508, Ph: 610-582-5571, email: rcaccese@talon.net).

McAll, K. (1982). *Healing the Family Tree.* London: Sheldon Press.

McAll, K. (1989). *Healing the Haunted.* London: Darley Anderson.

McAll, K. (1984). "Intercessory prayer format: Prayers for departed souls during Eucharistic liturgy." *Journal of Christian Healing 6(1)*: 45-46.

McAll, K (1993). "North American allergies: Healing Native American and settler legacies." *Journal of Christian Healing, 15(4):* 10-14.

McAll. K. (1983). "Ritual mourning in Anorexia Nervosa." *Journal of Christian Healing, 5(1):* 24-27.

Prince, D. (1990). *Blessing or Curse: You Can Choose.* Grand Rapids, MI: Chosen Books.

Schoeninger, D.W. (1988). "Tending family roots part 1: Foundational concepts." *Journal of Christian Healing, 10(1):* 22-28.

Schoeninger, D.W. (1989). "Tending family roots part II: Engaging the resources of our family legacy." *Journal of Christian Healing, 11(4):* 3-12.

Schoeninger, D.W. and Schoeninger, F. "Tending family roots part 3: Healing inherited tendencies." *Journal of Christian Healing, 16(2):* 3-15.

Sheldrake, R. (1988). *The Presence of the Past.* New York: Random House.

Smith, P. (1992). "Healing of generations: An ancient connection." *Journal of Christian Healing, 14(4):* 3-10.

Smith, P. (1996). *From Generation to Generation: A Manual for Healing.* Jacksonville, FL: Jahovah Rapha Press, P.O. Box 14780, Jacksonville, FL 32238-1470.

Taylor, Michael J. (1998). *Purgatory.* Huntington, IN: Our Sunday Visitor, Inc.

Chapter 14

Forgiveness and Healing the Repetition Compulsion

Charles Zeiders, Psy.D.
Julie Wegryn, M.A.
Christian Counseling and
Therapy Associates of Havertown
86 W Eagle Road
Havertown, PA 19083

Practitioners

Charles Zeiders, Psy.D., earned his Masters Degree in Counseling from Villanova University and his Doctorate in Clinical Psychology from Immaculata College. After his Postdoctoral Fellowship at the Center for Cognitive Therapy at the University of Pennsylvania in Philadelphia, he became Clinical Coordinator of Christian Counseling and Therapy Associates of Havertown. Topics of his publications include prayer and science, energy medicine, and the psychology of religion. He is a licensed psychologist and a Diplomate of Cognitive-Behavioral Psychology.

Julie Wegryn, M.A.T., M.S., NBCC earned her Masters Degree in Counseling from Villanova University. She serves on the Board of the Institute for Christian Counseling and Therapy and is Director of Christian Counseling and Therapy Associates of Havertown. She integrates Jungian psychology with healing prayer in her work as a Christian depth psychologist. She is a licensed psychologist and a Board Certified Counselor.

Introduction

The introduction of forgiveness to clients is among the most powerful interventions available to the Christian therapist. Over and over we find that our clients heal quickly and decisively, even of long-standing psychological wounds, when the prayer of forgiveness precedes the prayer for healing. We find that when our clients, using their free will in accordance with the teachings of Jesus of Nazareth, forgive those who trespass against them, then the psychological wounds sustained from those trespasses are made readily available to the healing power of God. This happens because forgiveness removes the barrier of unforgiveness that locks out God's healing grace. Because so many people enter into an experience of new life and rise to new levels of psychological wholeness following this particular prayer intervention, we believe that an extreme experience of renewed happiness is an effect of forgiveness. We call this the *Resurrection Effect*. Replacing the *Will to Punish* with the *Will to Forgive* is very good psychology and releases the *Resurrection Effect*.

Context

The authors worked as co-therapists with a 71 year old married Protestant woman, Loretta. She contacted Christian Counseling and Therapy Associates because she desired psychological treatment that included Christian healing practices.

Goal

As long as she could remember, Loretta experienced herself as a caregiver in her primary relationships. In the course of these relationships she found herself in a repeated pattern: She assumed an overly responsible role for others, slavishly expending herself on their behalf, but ultimately finding herself denigrated by those for whom she cared. As a result, she suffered from depression and emptiness, but she felt unable to escape from these painful relationships. She complained of having few friends, only people for whom she was responsible. Lastly, pain in her right leg, explained away as arthritic, added chronic pain to her experience of unhappiness. Treatment commenced with three goals:

1. Reduce depression and emptiness.
2. Reduce the frequency of the compulsively repeated care-until-rejected dynamic.
3. Develop friendships characterized by reciprocity instead of care-giving.

Case Illustration

Client History: Familial and Psychological Dynamics

We began co-therapy with Loretta. We met one time per week for six months. Some Cognitive-Behavioral interventions were offered, but we also engaged in psychodynamic-style uncovering. Once her story was told, we brainstormed as to how the forgiveness prayer might help her. Eventually, treatment culminated in the forgiveness prayer. We offered prayers throughout therapy and conducted all interventions in the name of Jesus Christ.

Family-of-origin issues formed the *Core Wound* that set forth so much unhappiness in her life. (A *Core Wound* can be thought of as a wound that is central to our very being and manifests as an empty, shattered place in the soul.) Her father was a highly placed official in a religious denomination. In early memories, Loretta recollects him admonishing that God's will for her life was to serve the nuclear family. God expected her, he told her, to put herself last and to take care of her mother and her two younger brothers. Fearing her father's and God's punishment if she disobeyed, she became *good* as good had been inflicted upon her. Instead of loving her in a way that would invigorate the core of her psyche with energy, her father abandoned that part of her to emptiness and indoctrinated her to a life of slavish service to her family.

Her mother played a similar role. Physically frail, lazy, and hypochondriacal, Loretta's mother never expended herself to praise Loretta. Rather, she sought to draw love, nurturing, and reassurance from Loretta, using her alleged sicknesses as the excuse for demanding that Loretta *mother* her. At one point, she told Loretta that unless Loretta fully obeyed her mother, her mother might become so upset that she would die. Hence, Loretta associated any demands she might make on her mother - whether through disobedience or asking for nurturing - as threats to her mother's life.

Both parents insisted that Loretta take parental-like responsibility for her younger brothers. This role as pseudo-parent set forth an ongoing childhood nightmare for Loretta. The younger brothers intuitively understood that although Loretta had responsibility for them, she had no authority over them. Their sadism caused them to delight in setting her up to fail.

On Sundays, Loretta had to prepare her little brothers for church. Her father made it clear that this chore was one of her Christian duties. Not to fulfill it would let God down and open her to verbal abuse and rejecting *guilt tripping* by her religious father. Her mother made it clear that she herself was too frail to dress the boys. Loretta had to dress them to prevent her mother from exhaustion. Under such pressure, Loretta would try to dress her little brothers. She would lay out their clothes and ask them to get dressed for church. Invariably, they would refuse to dress, throwing their clothes out windows and screaming when Loretta tried to correct them. They would run to the parents and accuse Loretta of wild injustice toward them. Loretta's father would blame and shame her for her failure to carry out God's work with her little brothers. Her mother would swoon, look troubled and frail, declaring that Loretta would be the death of her.

This family dynamic repeated itself throughout Loretta's childhood, adolescence, and adulthood. She recalled times that her brothers made poor investments. It then fell to her to give them money. They asked for loans as though they were entitled to them, but never repaid Loretta. At other times, when they needed advice, they never thanked her for good outcomes. When they thought that her advice was poor they denigrated her relentlessly.

When Loretta was a young mother involved in caring for her little children, she received a call from her youngest brother. He demanded that Loretta drop everything and immediately fly to the city where his wife was giving birth to their first child. Loretta was the only one, he exclaimed, who knew how to take care of children. At great personal sacrifice, Loretta honored her brother's request. She bundled up her infant children. She bought plane tickets. And, because her husband had to work, she flew alone to her brother and sister-in-law's to help them with their new infant. When she arrived, she found them very stressed from the new responsibility of parenthood. Despite her kindness, they scapegoated her for not arriving even sooner to help them. They also established humiliating house rules to which they told Loretta she would have to abide. Even in the face of their meanness, Loretta helped her nervous brother and sister-in-law. She helped them tremendously and selflessly, but they never thanked her. Even after their children were grown, they would allude to Loretta's visit as though she had done something slightly wrong to them.

Fortunately, Loretta married a kind, supportive man. He sought the best for his wife. He encouraged her to make friends outside of her family. He hoped that the establishment of a positive peer group would help Loretta find happier relationships. Unfortunately, this was not the case. Loretta found herself in relational dynamics very similar to the dynamics she experienced in her family-of-origin. For example, she reached out to a group of ladies in her church. At first, she got along well with them. So well, in fact, that they elected her to become the head of the growth committee. Then similar dynamics unfolded that reiterated the dynamics of her excruciating childhood Sunday mornings trying to dress her brothers. The church growth committee loaded Loretta with great responsibility but they provided her with little authority. When Loretta tried to make necessary changes, her *friends* on the committee rebelled and went to the pastor, complaining that Loretta was unreasonable. In turn, the pastor *guilt tripped* Loretta and told her that she would be the death of the church.

Listening to Loretta tell the story of these experiences, we learned of the emotional toll that was taken on her. For long periods throughout her life, she experienced a depressive emptiness at the core of her being. Also, much of the time she felt shame, as though there was something intrinsically wrong with her. She also had a vague awareness that her relations with her brothers were not right, but she could not help herself from getting into the same humiliating relations with them over and over. Lastly, despite her good marriage, she felt very lonely for a friend. All this emotional and relational pain was exacerbated by progressively debilitating leg pain that doctors attributed to arthritis.

Loretta told these things to us in treatment and our hearts went out to her. We conducted treatment and prayed. We developed a passion to understand the deep structure of her woundedness and to look to God for help in healing Loretta.

As Loretta's story unfolded, we found the following structure within her woundedness: From the beginning her parents rejected her. Obsessed with making Loretta do the *right* and *Christian* thing, Loretta's father had neglected to love his daughter. Similarly, Loretta's mother, neurotically striving to avoid her maternal responsibilities, used her hypochondriacal defenses to shirk her role as a nurturer. She forced Loretta to raise herself and her little brothers. She forced Loretta's compliance by telling Loretta that noncompliance with the situation would kill her. Instead of loving Loretta, both parents abandoned her. When children are abandoned, they often grow into adults who experience emptiness at the core. This was Loretta's case. She also felt anger for being sinned against by her parents, but she had to bring the anger back upon herself, because she had been indoctrinated that anger at her parents - and the *Will to Punish* that naturally arises from it - made her *bad* to her father and *murderous* to her mother. By turning such vitality - the vitality of anger - back upon herself she developed depression within her emptiness.

Next, the relationship her parents forced her to have with her brothers was especially damaging. Loretta was told that she had to meet the needs of her unappreciative brothers. In this way, she could be good in her father's eyes and keep her mother alive. Because her father's approval and her mother's life were contingent upon Loretta serving her sadistic, immature brothers, this relationship style became the only way that Loretta learned to relate to others. It followed her throughout her life. Each time Loretta repeated this relational dynamic, she experienced another wound that exacerbated the pain in her core. This repetition compulsion even influenced her relationship with the church growth committee and her pastor. She was compelled to repeat the relational dynamics of her childhood. In all these experiences, the lovelessness of the relational dynamics kept her core empty and the anger she turned back upon herself kept her in a state of depression. (Loretta agreed with these interpretations. They modeled reality as she understood it. All of us agreed, however, that only God sees the entire picture, and that none of us really understood the moral or spiritual nature of those who had hurt Loretta in an ultimate sense. God, not ourselves, is the final authority.)

Specific Healing Interventions

Loretta wanted to be free from wounded painful relationships. To meet her need, we discussed Jesus' teaching regarding how unforgiveness locks in our woundedness and how forgiveness frees us for healing. We further proposed that we had gathered enough information about Loretta's past to move to the next decisive stage of healing: the forgiveness prayer. Anxious to heal, Loretta readily agreed.

We opened the prayer in Jesus' name. Then we approached God with the prayer intention that God would heal Loretta from the emptiness and depression she felt and that he would free her from the abusive relational dynamics that plagued her. Recalling, however, that Loretta had outstanding business with those who had trespassed against her, we left these prayer intentions for healing and went to the place within her where she maintained the *Will to Punish* her father. She replaced her *Will to Punish* him for indoctrinating her to be the family slave with the *Will to Forgive* him for this sin against her. She did the same thing with her mother for not nurturing her and for forcing her to take over the role of mother to her brothers. She then forgave her brothers for the way they wounded her by abusing her nurturing and for their sadism and lack of appreciation. She then began to replace the *Will to Punish* with the *Will to Forgive* regarding other people in her life with whom she had experienced similar hurtful dynamics - including the ladies from the church growth committee and her pastor. Still in prayer, we returned to the original prayer intention. Having forgiven those who trespassed against her, Loretta had, by using her free *Will to Forgive*, freed herself from the unforgiveness that blocked out the healing power of the Holy Spirit from the wounds that others had inflicted upon her. We acknowledged that Loretta had forgiven others their failings, just as Jesus had taught. We asked God to now heal Loretta of the way those failings had harmed her soul.

When we concluded this prayer, it was obvious that the clinical situation had entered into a state of unusual grace. The feeling of joy and energy that accompanies the special presence of the Holy Spirit permeated our office. Loretta left feeling encouraged. Immediately, she began using the forgiveness prayer. On her drive home, she reported, she had the impression that the Holy Spirit was bringing different people to mind who had injured her psyche. In prayer, she replaced her *Will to Punish* these people with the *Will to Forgive* them. Then she asked the Father in Jesus' name to send the Holy Spirit to heal the part of her soul that had sustained damage from those who had sinned against her.

Therapeutic Process

By this time, Loretta had been in therapy for six months. Within four months she had finished the bulk of stage one, the stage of problem definition. In less than a month, she finished stage two, the stage of developing an intellectual understanding of how forgiving her trespassers could lead to healing. The rest of her sessions were spent praying the forgiveness prayer and discussing outcomes. The outcomes themselves were staggering. Within a very short period of time, Loretta experienced a radical decrease in her experience of inner emptiness and depression. Within five weeks of practicing the forgiveness prayer, Loretta noticed that she had not experienced her repetition compulsion. She found that in none of her relationships had she fallen into the care-take-until-abuse dynamic that plagued and hurt her throughout her life. Following her forgiveness work, she developed a spontaneous ability to avoid the old dynamic and to draw boundaries. She delighted in suddenly finding herself appropriately assertive. Further, just following her forgiveness work, she began a friendship with a woman in her church. Loretta found the experience of friendship delightful. Rather than giving to another while waiting to be abused, Loretta had the first intimate relationship with another person (outside her marriage) that was characterized by respect and reciprocity. Finally, the pain Loretta had in her leg - originally attributed to arthritis - diminished by 85%, according to Loretta's self-report. All these breakthroughs occurred following the initial forgiveness prayer and Loretta's ongoing discipline of practicing it.

Because Loretta experienced such profound relief and experienced a welcome elevation to an energized sense of well being, she was a beneficiary of the *Resurrection Effect* of Forgiveness.

Psychological Theory

When a person, like Loretta, feels trapped in a painful relationship style, we begin to think that something went wrong in childhood and has continued into adulthood. Maybe the parents were overly involved. Maybe they were not involved enough. Maybe the parents put unreasonable demands on the child. Maybe the child was especially sensitive and just plain prone to being wounded. What is clear is that something went wrong and the child was hurt. When the hurt is deep, we call it a *Core Wound*. A *Core Wound* can be thought of as an empty, shattered place in the soul. Around that shattered place, anger accumulates. Anger gives rise to a *Will to Punish*. The *Will to Punish* is connected to ideas like, "I was hurt and I won't be satisfied until someone is punished." Sometimes, people override their anger and try to gain the approval of the people who hurt them. They think, "If I please them, then they will love me, and I will not be hurt anymore." Some individuals go through life compelled to enter relationships that repeatedly hurt them, hoping that their *Core Wound*, anger, and the *Will to Punish* will relent, if they gain the approval of those who hurt them. We call this the repetition compulsion.

Theology

The teachings of Jesus of Nazareth inform the psychology of healing *Core Wounds* and related problems. In this regard, Our Lord's teachings from Mt. 5: 21-26 are immeasurably helpful. Jesus teaches how our psychological responses to others' trespasses against us, cause us to inadvertently construct psychological prisons for ourselves that lock us into those wounds. Jesus tells us that when someone hurts us, we experience them as a *Traitor* or a *Fool*. Having others betray us or treat us foolishly hurts us psychologically. For example, when a parent betrays a child by withholding love, the wound of emptiness inflicted on the child's core will cause the child to see that parent as a *Traitor*.

From the *Core Wound,* a feeling of anger at the meanness and injustice, the betrayal or hurtful foolishness, emerges. Anger radiates from the *Core Wound* and an intention to punish the offenders develops. In our practical theology, we call this desire the *Will to Punish*. It is a natural response to others who sin against us. Yet, this natural response, this *Will to Punish*, also traps the wound into our psychic structures. Jesus explains it this way,

> Anyone who is angry with a brother will answer for it before the court; and anyone who calls a brother "Fool" will answer for it before the Sanhedrin; and anyone who calls him "Traitor" will answer for it in hellfire (Mt. 5:22-23).

Others make us angry, Jesus teaches, because they treat us in a sinful way. Yet, when we develop a *Will to Punish* them as they have punished us, we imprison ourselves in unforgiveness. When we want to punish others for the sins they commit against us, it is as though our own *Will to Punish* becomes a prison that locks out God's healing grace from the hurt within our soul, while imprisoning the wound itself in the core of our psyche.

In the example of the child who suffers the parental treason of neglect or abuse, a *Will to Punish* the offending parent will harm the child's ability to heal from the parent's sin. The *Will to Punish* the offending parent locks in the wound of painful lovelessness and the painful anger at the injustice. At the same time, the *Will to Punish* will also lock out God's healing grace that would restore love to the child's core and thus heal the wound.

Fortunately, Jesus teaches how to heal. Healing the psychological wound involves replacing the *Will to Punish* with the *Will to Forgive*. Jesus teaches us to forgive others their failings when we stand in prayer, so that our Father in heaven will forgive us our failings (Mk. 11:25). If we think of our failings as anything outside the perfect will of God for our psyche, we see that forgiving others for trespassing against us helps God to heal us of the failings they inflicted upon us. In other words, replacing the *Will to Punish* with the *Will to Forgive* removes the psychological barrier of unforgiveness and allows God's grace to heal us of our wounds. Jesus gets us out of prison, and he snatches us from hellfire. By forgiving, we create the psychological condition that allows God to restore our soul.

Importantly, the Kingdom of God is predicated on free *Will*. We do not have to forgive others unless we wish. Replacing the *Will to Punish* with the *Will to Forgive* amounts to an act of will - an ego intention. When we approach God to pray for healing of our of wounds, we know that something is required of our *Will* before our prayer for inner healing will be effective. We intend that those who caused us to suffer will not owe us the debt of similar suffering. We willfully stop requiring that those we want to punish will be punished. Seeing us employ our *Will* in this way, God heals us of the wound inflicted on us by the Traitors and Fools we forgive. In Matthew 5:23-24, Jesus teaches,

> If you are bringing your offering to the altar and there remember that your brother has something against you, leave your offering there before the altar, go and be reconciled with your brother first, and then come back and present your offering.

Jesus gives us a allegory for how to use our ego intentions to be blessed by the Father's healing grace. Only God can heal the psyche. Over that we have no control. Yet, we do have the freedom to forgive those who wounded our psyche in the first place. When we use our freedom to forgive those who sin against us, God then uses his grace to heal the psychological wounds that they inflicted upon us.

Methodology
The clinical process that leads to forgiveness and eventual healing has three stages:
1. problem definition
2. psycho-spiritual education, and
3. healing prayer

The first stage involves defining the problem. This stage involves establishing who hurt the client, how they were hurt, and how the hurt established a painful psychological pattern. This stage also identifies that someone sinned against the client and hurt them. This stage concludes when the client's anger is available to the ego.

The second stage pivots the client's awareness from how they were wounded to how Jesus' teaching about forgiveness offers them the opportunity to heal. During this stage of treatment, the therapist shows how relevant teachings from Matthew 5 pertain directly to the client's issues.

The third stage involves helping the client pray a prayer of forgiveness for the hurts inflicted upon them by Traitors and Fools; then, with the *Will to Punish* no longer blocking God's grace, client and therapist pray for the healing of the wound inflicted by those trespassers upon the psyche.

Treatment involves the therapist leading the client in a variation of the following prayer:

Father, I pray in Jesus' name and according to his teachings. I have a wound inside my soul. It is my intention to offer a prayer for healing of that wound. But Jesus told me to make peace with those who inflicted this wound upon me before I offer this prayer. When I freely offer forgiveness to those who have hurt me, when I replace my *Will to Punish* with my *Will to Forgive*, then I free this inflicted wound from the prison of unforgiveness. Then my wound is free to experience your healing grace and no barrier exists within me that locks out your restorative goodness.

Thus, Father, in Jesus' name, I will ask you to heal the wound that _____ inflicted upon me. But, I leave my prayer intention like an offering at your altar. I go to that place in me where I see _____, who hurt me through the following act of Treason and/or Foolishness _____. Even though they wronged me, I seek to follow the teachings of your son, Jesus Christ. Using my free *Will*, I excuse them of any obligation to me. I no longer require that they experience a punishment like the one they inflicted upon me. I replace my *Will to Punish* them with a *Will to Forgive* them.

Now that I have made peace with those who hurt me, God, I return to my prayer intention like a person returning to your altar after making peace with his brother. Lord God, I continue to pray in Jesus' name that you will heal the wound inflicted on me by those I just forgave. I have forgiven them their failings.

Please heal me of the way their failings have damaged my soul. Please take away the absence-of-love, the anger, the anxiety, the shame, the pain, the deep hurt. Please heal painful ways of relating that spring from this wound. Please restore the Image of God to that part of my soul. Thank you for sending the Holy Spirit with your healing grace. In Jesus' name. Amen.

Conclusion

When others trespass against us we can develop *Core Wounds*. Around these *Core Wounds* anger develops and gives rise to the *Will to Punish* those who hurt us. We also develop dysfunctional coping behaviors. By following Jesus' teaching on forgiveness we can heal. By replacing the *Will to Punish* our trespassers with the *Will to Forgive* them, our *Core Wounds* become available to God's healing grace. When God heals us, we experience a sense of new life so great, we call it the *Resurrection Effect*. Following Loretta's replacement of the *Will to Punish* with the *Will to Forgive*, God blessed Loretta with healing and the *Resurrection Effect*. God will do the same for us and for our patients.

Spiritual Direction and Prayer Ministry

Chapter 15

A Generational Nightmare

Louis Lussier, O.S.Cam., M.D., Ph.D.
3661 S Kinnickinnic Ave.
St. Francis, WI 53235

Practitioner

Louis Lussier, O.S.Cam., M.Div., M.D., Ph.D., graduated from the University of Montreal Medical School in 1969; he obtained his Ph.D. from Penn State University in Applied (Exercise) Physiology in 1978; he received an M.Div. from Sacred Heart School of Theology in 1990. He completed his training in Physical Medicine and Rehabilitation in 1978 and is Board certified in Canada and the USA.

Training and Journey of Integration
Through my medical and theological studies and my involvement with healing prayer - receiving it personally and ministering it - I began to see the human person as much more than my studies had led me to recognize. The profound unity of the person in health and disease intrigued me. As I discovered the generational dimension, I added a new perspective to that unity and explored though this ministry the influence of the spiritual realm on human existence.

Context

The context of this illustration is a generational healing ministry conducted with a team of persons who pray using the gifts of the Holy Spirit, particularly gifts of knowledge and discernment of spirits. A team member's employee brought to the team's attention the story of her husband. This was shared with the team at a conference where we had gathered; we prayed for clarity. I met the man twice and, with the team, provided the ministry he needed. Later I met with his wife (the employee); this led to more ministry.

Goal

The goal of ministry was to free the man from nightmares and pray for the healing of the wife's deceased father.

Theory/Theology/Scripture

The concept of the journey of life is central to the understanding of this

---

* First published in *The Journal of Christian Healing*, Volume 20, Number 3&4, Fall/Winter, 1998, pp. 86-93.

story. Our journey appears to be completed after death should we not resolve our conflicts and divisions during our lifetime or die with wounds never opened to healing: "If your brother has something against you ... I warn you, you will not be released until you have paid the last penny (Mt. 5:23-26)." The gospels tell us that life's journey is focused on relationships and love, on community and reconciliation. Life's goal is to surrender freely into the arms of God the Father, in a trusting and loving response. When a journey ends prematurely or uncompleted, a person may not be able to move into the divine embrace until the work of salvation is done: release from all that holds others and self in bondage. Living persons may reach out to their ancestors through intercessory prayer, forgiveness, and Eucharist. The power of the love expressed by the living becomes a catalyst, a jumpstart, to turn ancestors who are trapped and chained (like Jacob Marley in Dickens *A Christmas Carol*). The living can help them build trust and hope where before there was resistance to continue the journey into new life. We witness to those who have died as to our faith in the gospel we have received (I Pet 3:18-4:6).

Methodology
1. Research the family history and develop the family tree.
2. Pray with the gifts of the Spirit to uncover facts or "myths" to better understands the issues.
3. Pray to break the bondages, curses, dedications, and to deliver from demonic strongholds.
4. Celebrate Eucharist to invite the departed ancestors to enter the heavenly banquet.

Case History
M. had been in law enforcement for many years and had given little attention to his spiritual walk for most of his life. Though baptized in the Roman Catholic Church, he was notably influenced by his maternal grandfather who drank alcohol heavily, gambled, and got into fights, ending up in jail. This grandfather, Catholic in name only, raised M. M's maternal grandmother died young, when M. was four or five years of age.

M's father was promiscuous and never could be found at home. Consequently M. never felt any closeness to him. As a teen M. went to bars with his father and got drunk. M's parents divorced when M. was a marine and he had rarely seen his father since. M's father abandoned his young daughter and she lives a life much like her father. M's mother is both passive and controlling. She presently suffers from heart disease.

M's paternal grandmother was a greedy, mean and self-centered woman, who lost her husband early in the marriage and was left with five boys and without support. Her husband, who died of a heart attack, was a preacher.

M. married at the age of 19. The marriage lasted three years. His wife was into parties, prostitution, drugs and jail. She was beaten to death by her boyfriend some time after the divorce. M. remarried and with his present wife G., has a stable marriage. M. had dated G. several times as a teenager. He had briefly met her father three times. He began to rekindle the relationship with G. three years after her father died. They now have a daughter and have adopted M's nephew.

In January 1997, M. began to have weird dreams. In the dreams he observed himself dying in a different way every night - car accident, shooting, stabbing, falling off a building, drowning …. This was followed for the next two weeks by dreams of being dead and lying in a casket. The casket was in a room with no lights or color, just grayness or blackness without walls. People mingled around conversing. M. did not recognize anyone nor could he understand the conversations.

About a month after the onset of the dreams, M. recognized five persons around the casket: his maternal grandfather who died of a heart attack in 1978, the one who had raised him; his ex-wife who had died in 1992; his cousin Jackie, who was a marine, an alcoholic, a nominal Catholic and who had shot himself in the head in 1992; his father-in law (G's father) who died in 1977; and a mystery marine in a WW II uniform. These people walked by the casket, talked to him and asked questions. M. could not open his eyes or speak but saw all this as though he were watching television.

After a few weeks of this form of nightmare, a priest-like figure stood over him and delivered a eulogy, emphasizing his good deeds and remaining quiet about his sins. Finally he realized that the five people were burying him since he heard dirt hitting the casket. M. thought that this would be the end of the dreams and they ceased for three or four nights. Then the nightmares recurred and he found himself tearing the bed apart as he tried to get out of the tomb. This lasted a week. Then part of the group of five visitors dug him up, dragged him into the same room where he had been waked. They opened the casket and proceeded to tell him why he was there. They foretold that M. would have a violent, near-death experience and that it would be up to him to choose to survive it. He was told that his time had not yet come and he was to gather his strength for the struggle.

After a few more weeks, in the dreams, his grandfather affirmed M. and his family and told M. that he was proud of him, assuring him that all would be well. Then he left the room and did not return. His ex-wife told him that she did not want to see him again and left. His father-in-law also assured him that things would go well and left. As they exited, M. described them as looking terrible, deadlike, while they had looked fine previously.

M's cousin Jackie and the old marine did not speak to him but remained in the room. Then someone entered to torture him while he still lay in the casket. The old marine did nothing while Jackie laughed at his pain. The torturer had very cold hands, stuck ice picks in both M's temples, and pulled out his fingernails (much like prisoner of war tortures).

The nightmares were continuing when I met with M. in May, 1997. He could barely sleep anymore in order to avoid the nightmares. M's wife G. reported that she had asked M. specifically what her father had said to him. She realized that her father had revealed things that M. had no possibility of knowing, things she herself had forgotten. They both felt that five deceased persons from his past were visiting M. during these nightmares. After my interview with M., I felt that this was an intergenerational event and would approach it as such.

The team began to pray for the Holy Spirit's guidance. Masonic influence on the family was identified. The history of military involvement was also studied. M. remembered an uncle who had died during the second world war after suffering a neck wound at the age of 19. He was transported on a hospital ship that was sunk by a Japanese submarine. He died along with all the other passengers and crew. M. also pointed out that some of his ancestry came from pre Civil War Missouri in times of division affecting whole families.

In June 1997, we gathered for the celebration of the Eucharist for M's family. We prayed to break the bondage of Freemasonry on the family and prayed for forgiveness of all the hatred and division within the family. We felt strongly that the family had been divided over the slavery issue with members fighting on both sides of the Civil War and with the possibility of fratricide during that conflict. The matriarch had experienced a deeply broken heart. This fact seemed related to a prevalence of premature deaths from heart disease in women of this ancestry. Also the family division was reflected in the history of abandonment of children with three generations affected within memory. This was all brought to the altar for prayer, healing and reconciliation.

We prayed that the family would be freed of all demonic assignments and guardians of the bondages. We asked forgiveness specifically for the sins of the ex-wife and the cousin. We prayed that the five visitors would embrace the salvation that Jesus had merited for them. As the Spirit led us, we prayed for any who had been hurt by the family's sins. One member of the group had a vision of the ancestor who was a Mason, sobbing and repenting. M. repented in the name of his family and ancestors. We could sense spiritual heaviness lift progressively as forgiveness flowed and bondages were broken.

Following the Mass, M had several dreams with the original cast of characters. In the dreams he was no longer dead in the casket but he was still apart from them. However, the dreams were no longer menacing. In one dream, the older marine, now identified as his uncle killed in WW II, was ready to move on and thanked him. His ex-wife also came to thank him. His cousin Jackie berated him for meddling with his fate and left. His grandfather, the most supportive also moved on after arguing with the father-in-law who blamed everyone for his ills and judged everyone. In the dreams, the father-in-law had expressed disapproval toward M. as his son-in-law. M., himself, now confronted him and the father-in-law left.

M. began to experience deep and peaceful sleep at this point. He had undergone a change of heart, beginning with a new relationship with Jesus Christ. He has since moved out of law enforcement.

The issue of the *father-in-law* was affecting G., M's wife. We looked into the family history of this man, the son of a converted moonshiner who became a Pentecostal minister. G's dad was the oldest of ten children and was afflicted with a congenital heart and lung disease. He suffered his first heart attack at the age of 28 years and became a cardiac invalid. He ruled his family as a paranoid dictator, carrying a gun on him out of fear. He died at 40 years of age, angry that God had not responded to all the prayers for healing solicited by his father.

This situation was first addressed in a prayer session in December 1997. Forgiveness and release of her father was prayed through by G. who carried a lot of heaviness in her heart. She often had sensed a presence around her as though living in a haunted house. Mass was celebrated in April, 1998. We prayed for all ethnic conflict within the family, since there is a Native American root in the family tree. We asked the Lord for a new heart for G's dad and for his release from the bondage of bitterness, anger and distrust, as evidenced by his accusations and resentment toward M., in the dreams. We received a strong sense that this man being stripped of his tattered suit and was clothed in the garment of salvation.

In July, 1998, I had the opportunity to visit with G. She told me that since the Mass, she had felt a deep sense of release, no disturbing presence around her, and a peace about her dad. M. has continued to sleep soundly and experiences a new lease on life.

Discussion

People have different views of what happens to individuals after death. If we accept this story, our preconceptions are shaken, especially as we suspect that things may not be as we envisioned them. Our views on life after death may prevent us from reaching out to those calling for help by denying that they are in a state of unrest. Stories of hauntings and visitations have been around for centuries and are ridiculed today as not scientifically verifiable. Much of this has been relegated to the field of the paranormal. However, these manifestations of the spiritual realm respond to prayer and Eucharist.

The ministry of generational healing has provided me with a new understanding of *purgatory*. As I see it now, purgatory appears to be a place where we work out what is in need of reconciliation, of liberation from bondage; where we begin to turn our face toward God and experience God's loving gaze. It is a place to complete our journey, to become unstuck from the traps we created by sin, by the wounding of others, by our refusal of God's call and God's love. It requires a choice to engage anew the journey into freedom, into God's salvation for us. A stuck soul may need the love of descendants to help and support him/her in making that choice. This love of the descendants is best expressed in intercessory prayer and the Eucharist.

As a team prays through a generational situation, they often get a *scenario*, a story of things that may have occurred. Questions are asked about the historicity of this *scenario*, particularly when it goes far back in the history of the family and is unverifiable. I believe that this *scenario* is given to direct our prayer, rather than give us historical facts. I believe it has a solid base in truth but details may not be accurate. When the situation is contemporary, I have found the knowledge received through discerning prayer to be accurate.

Curses also are real and result from our actions as much as from our words and rituals. In this story, the feud between brothers left the family cursed with division, abandonment, and broken hearts in mothers for generations. Scripture tells us that actions that disregard God's word to us bring upon us a curse, inherent to turning away from God (Deut. 28:15-69). On the other hand, obedience to God's word is rewarded with blessings (Deut. 28:1-14).

As I continue in this ministry, I receive a clearer vision of God's salvific activity. This is different from the paranormal which generally studies such events as isolated and curious. I believe we are part of a large pilgrimage and along the way we help one another and we hurt one another; we urge one another on or we impede one another's progress. Death modifies our existence, but the pilgrimage continues. Anyone who is stuck because he/she is not ready to die may need help to accept the grace he/she refused in this life. Hell could be seen as a choice to remain permanently stuck in anger, hatred, fear, ... sin. Generational healing helps both the living and the dead to continue the journey.

References

Boszormenyi-Nagy, I., and Krasner, B. R. (1986). *Between Give and Take. A Clinical Guide to Contextual Therapy.* New York: Brunner/Mazel.

Boszormenyi-Nagy, I., and Spark, G.M. (1973). *Invisible Loyalties: Reciprocity in Intergenerational Family Therapy.* New York: Harper and Row.

Epstein, A.W. (1982). "Mental phenomena across generations: The holocaust," *Journal of the American Academy of Psychoanalysis. 10, 565-570.*

Fiore, E. (1987). *The Unquiet Dead.* New York: Ballantine Books.

Hampsch, J.H. (1986). *Healing Your Family Tree.* Everett, WA: Performance Press.

Linn, M., Linn, D. and Fabricant S. (1985). *Healing the Greatest Hurt.* Mahwah, NJ: Paulist Press.

McAll, K. (1992) *Conference on Healing the Family Tree.* West Chester, PA: Institute for Christian Counseling and Therapy (ICCT), set of ten audio tapes including prayers for departed ancestors (for a complete list of audio and video offerings on Generational Healing and other topics of Christian Healing from ICCT contact: Robin Caccese, 137 Proudfoot Drive, Birdsboro, PA 19508, Ph: 610-582-5571, email: rcaccese@talon.net).

McAll, K. (1982). *Healing the Family Tree.* London: Sheldon Press.

McAll, K. (1989). *Healing the Haunted.* London: Darley Anderson.

McAll, K. (1984). "Intercessory prayer format: Prayers for departed souls during Eucharistic liturgy." *Journal of Christian Healing. 6(1):* 45-46.

McAll, K (1993). "North American allergies: Healing Native American and settler legacies." *Journal of Christian Healing. 15(4):* 10-14.

McAll. K. (1983). "Ritual mourning in Anorexia Nervosa." *Journal of Christian Healing. 5(1):* 24-27.

Prince, D. (1990). *Blessing or Curse: You Can Choose.* Grand Rapids, MI: Chosen Books.

Schoeninger, D.W. (1988). "Tending family roots part 1: Foundational concepts." *Journal of Christian Healing. 10(1):* 22-28.

Schoeninger, D.W. (1989). "Tending family roots part II: Engaging the resources of our family legacy." *Journal of Christian Healing. 11(4):* 3-12.

Schoeninger, D.W. and Schoeninger, F. "Tending family roots part 3: Healing inherited tendencies." *Journal of Christian Healing. 16(2):* 3-15.

Sheldrake, R. (1988). *The Presence of the Past.* New York: Random House.

Smith, P. (1992). "Healing of generations: An ancient connection." *Journal of Christian Healing. 14(4):* 3-10.

Smith, P. (1996). *From Generation to Generation: A Manual for Healing.* Jacksonville, FL: Jahovah Rapha Press, P.O. Box 14780, Jacksonville, FL 32238-1470.

Taylor, Michael J. (1998). *Purgatory.* Huntington, IN: Our Sunday Visitor, Inc.

Chapter 16

Jesus Christ The Ultimate Healer: Adult Children of the King (ACOK)

Robert McGuire, S.J., M.Th.
Spirit Life Center
300 Washington Ave.
Plainview, NY 11803

Practitioner:

Fr. Robert McGuire of the Society of Jesus is the Founder and Director of the Spirit Life Center and the ACOK (the Adult Child of the King) program. He is a native of New York City and was ordained in 1958. His initial ministry was as a Guidance Counselor at Regis High School, a Jesuit Scholarship school in Manhattan. After thirteen years of work with high school students he was baptized in the Spirit in 1972, and experienced a deep transformation and a new direction. He became a leader in the Catholic Charismatic Renewal and traveled to Japan, Korea, Israel, Yugoslavia, and Rome where he witnessed a tremendous upsurge of the Holy Spirit in Catholic and other Christian Churches.

Fr. McGuire was stationed at the St. Pius X House of Prayer in Plainview, New York from 1978-1991. He is currently Director of the Spirit Life Center. The Center is dedicated to Christ's healing ministry. Through the exercise of the gifts of the Holy Spirit, the Spirit Life Community has been able to bring a unique peace to the emotionally poor. Under the direction of Fr. McGuire the Spirit Life team has developed different outreach programs to Catholic parishes throughout Long Island and Queens called *The Quest*. This mission consists of a unique combination of preaching, liturgical dance, music and drama that culminates in a Healing Mass. As a speaker and Eucharist Celebrant, Fr. McGuire has traveled throughout the States, the British Virgin Islands, and most recently to Australia. He has lead pilgrimages around the world.

Fr. McGuire is also one of the founders of Resurrection Press, a Catholic Charismatic publishing company dedicated to the ministry of healing. In addition to running the different programs at the Spirit Life Center, Fr. McGuire is a member of the Association of Christian Therapists (ACT). Fr. McGuire and the Spirit Life Community represent a new approach to evangelization and the renewal of the Church.

The Story

In reality, this *Story* is *His Story*. This is Jesus' story of healing. In the summer of 1990 a group of 12 (in some way like the apostles) began to gather in a Catholic school to praise, to pray and to seek a deeper Christ-centered approach to inner healing and the 12-Steps. We were not sure where we were going but sure that we all wanted Jesus Christ to be our explicit guide as well as our Higher Power. All 12 in the group had been involved in Charismatic prayer meetings. We began to integrate prayer with songs of praise, scripture and petition. A fine book called *The Twelve Steps: A Spiritual Journey* (1994), became for us a working guide for adult children from addictive and other dysfunctional families. We became conscious at our weekly meetings that there was a gradual healing and integrating process going on within us. We moved purposefully through the 12-Steps and a format began to develop. There was a harmonization of the 12-Steps and the Catholic Charismatic Renewal. By the end of the first year we moved to the Spirit Life Center where by *word of mouth* other participants began to come and share. We now call this program ACOK.

As a confirmation of the fruitfulness of ACOK since its conception ten years ago, we have had almost 3,000 participants in the program. The counseling is existential. The larger expanse of Spirit Life is family related. The adult child is being nurtured again and is re *membered* into a healthier and wholistic life centered around Jesus Christ.

Context

ACOK is the basic expression of the Spirit Life vision. It is a faith community of worship journeying towards wholeness. It is a Catholic 12-Step program integrating prayer, scripture, and the sacraments with the format of the 12-Steps. The program, although Catholic, is open to all denominations provided they accept our Catholic identity and structure. It is in the true open Spirit of Vatican II. It is a special formative program whose members seek a deeper spiritual life as expressed in the 11th and 12th steps. It is complimentary to the regular 12-step programs, such as *A.A.* and *Alanon*. It is for the people who have overcome the struggle for abstinence and are now searching to deepen their spiritual life, mend relationships and strive for a better quality of living by changing their behavior and attitudes through the power of the Holy Spirit. Ideally speaking, the program should be linked to a full conversion through the Baptism in the Holy Spirit.

Program Goals
1. To integrate the recovery from addiction with a deeper conversion and with the formation of a strong spiritual life linked to the Catholic Church and for others to their own denomination.
2. To connect the ACOK 12-Step Program with the overall vision of the Spirit Life Center.

3. To facilitate healing from the trauma of childhood.
4. To assist those in the program to a closer relationship to community and to parish life.
5. To motivate the participants to a spirit of evangelization.

Theology

This program can be integrated with all the Catholic traditions linked to scripture, liturgy and spirituality. It also can be adapted to the other Christian Churches according to their traditions. The structure is developmental in accordance with the healing and conversion process of the individual. The following 12-steps are explicitly centered on Jesus Christ, the Church, and the Sacraments as the process towards wholeness.

The 12-Steps

Step One: We admitted we were powerless over the effects of our separation from God and that our lives have become unmanageable.

Step Two: Came to believe that a power, Jesus, who is greater than ourselves, could restore us to sanity.

Step Three: Made a decision to turn our will and our lives over to the care of God.

Step Four: Made a searching and fearless moral inventory of ourselves.

Step Five: Admitted to God, to ourselves, and to another human being the exact nature of our wrongs.

Step Six: We became entirely ready to have God remove all these defects of character.

Step Seven: Humbly asked God to remove all our shortcomings.

Step Eight: Made a list of all persons we had harmed and became willing to make amends.

Step Nine: Made direct amends to such people wherever possible, except when to do so would injure them or others.

Step Ten: Continued to take personal inventory and when wrong, promptly admit it.

Step Eleven: Sought, through prayer and meditation to improve our conscious contact with Jesus Christ, praying only for knowledge of his Will for us and the power to carry that out.

Step Twelve: Having had a spiritual awakening as the result of these steps, we tried to carry this message to others, and to practice these principles in all our affairs.

At Spirit Life we believe that healing can take place through a radical commitment to Jesus Christ and the sacraments in the Catholic Church. The universality of the 12-steps is be applied to the traditional spirituality of the

Church. This begins with a deep sense of prayer, repentance and reconciliation to the Lord. Step 4 is a moral inventory. It is synonymous with an examination of conscience. Step 5 should be linked to confession or a deep openness to a sponsor. In the light that Steps 6 through 10 are deeply linked to repentance, reconciliation and the mercy of Jesus Christ, a special Healing Mass along with the sacrament of the Anointing of the Sick can draw these steps together. Steps 11 and 12 should integrate the gifts of the Holy Spirit and a major commitment to scripture, liturgy and evangelization.

Theory
Good Spirituality is Good Therapy
Because of the trauma of the past, there is a radical need of healing and reconciliation. *We are what we remember, and more importantly, we are how we remember.* We need to understand why we have behaved in unhealthy, self-destructive ways. In an effort to understand ourselves better, ACOK members have become acquainted with many sound therapeutic concepts including the healing of the inner child through the recollection of memories and generational cleansing.

Each one of us carries the wounded child of our past. This child carries the memories and experiences of life. It is part of us that has not fully matured because we experienced trauma or deprivation during our developmental years. Although we have grown in many ways we are still lacking the wholeness that will bring peace.

We can learn to be re-parented and to nurture ourselves. We do this by facing our past and moving through the forgiveness process. We need a spirit of forgiveness for ourselves and others. We invite Jesus, who is Lord of the past, present and future to touch these painful memories and soften their hold on us. Then with an infilling of the Spirit, we can move on to a healthier, happier life closer to wholeness. This type of healing is a process. It is a way of life. The spiritual life of ACOK offers the experience of a loving positive environment and a family of faith.

Breaking the Cycle
The central theme of ACOK is related to the healing of the adult child within. The following are characteristic of the adult behavior that develops from alcoholism within the family. These characteristics are dealt within the ACOK program:
- Adult children of alcoholics guess at what normal is.
- Adult children of alcoholics have trouble following a project through from beginning to end.
- Adult children of alcoholics tell lies when it would be just as easy to tell the truth.

- Adult children of alcoholics judge themselves without mercy.
- Adult children of alcoholics have difficulty having fun.
- Adult children of alcoholics take themselves very seriously.
- Adult children of alcoholics have difficulty with intimate relationships.
- Adult children of alcoholics over react to changes over which they have no control.
- Adult children of alcoholics constantly seek approval and affirmation.
- Adult children of alcoholics usually feel different from other people.
- Adult children of alcoholics are super responsible or super-irresponsible.
- Adult children of alcoholics are extremely loyal, even in the face of evidence that the loyalty is undeserved.
- Adult children of alcoholics tend to lock themselves into a course of action without giving serious consideration to alternative behaviors or possible consequence. This impulsivity leads to confusion, self-loathing, and loss of control of the environment. As a result, they spend tremendous amounts of time *cleaning up the mess.*

Methodology

ACOK meets regularly on Friday evening. The people arrive at 7:30 p.m. and are greeted by a hospitality team. Everyone is given a name tag with their first name. Newcomers are encouraged to enroll in the program and given information on Spirit Life. A team consisting of facilitators encourages the people to sit before the Blessed Sacrament in the Spirit Life Chapel for half an hour of quiet prayer. Ideally, these facilitators should be in regular attendance at the meetings, should have the capacity for not only leadership, but for an in-depth understanding of the steps. The team meets from 7:30 p.m. to 8:00 p.m. for prayer, discernment and planning. At 8:00 p.m. there is a period of praise and song integrated with scriptural readings that are focused on the step of the night. An offering is taken up at this time to help sustain the program. A guest speaker speaks for 20 to 30 minutes on the step and their life conversion. As a guide for the speakers, the book *The Twelve Steps - A Spiritual Journey, a working guide for healing damaged emotions (based on biblical teachings)* is used. Each member of the ACOK program has their own copy of this book. This publication is made immediately available in the Spirit Life Bookstore.

After the talk the main facilitator of the evening divides the participants into small groups consisting of 5-8 people, depending on the number attending. Before meeting in their small groups, a 15-minute break with refreshments is provided. The groups then re-assemble. With an individual facilitator they share, anonymously, their story in accord with the talk and the step.

Newcomers are asked to meet in the Chapel where a chosen facilitator gives them an orientation on the program. Ideally, every member of the group should have a time to share. The groups meet for about 45 minutes. At the end of the small group sharing, the participants form a circle and recite a closing prayer, and each member is asked to pray during the week for the person on their right. A bell is then rung to bring all the people back together in the large group. The large group meets in the lounge for announcements. People are made aware of upcoming seminars, communion breakfasts, the ACOK (4th Friday of the month) Healing Mass, the monthly Charismatic Mass, weekly mini-retreat, women and men's spirituality events, café and prayer meeting. As preparation for the next week volunteers are asked to bring refreshments and supplies for the next meeting. The evening ends with a prayer and the ACOK theme song *I Believe* is sung.

After dismissal there may be time for individual consultation. Members are given the opportunity to go into the Spirit Life Bookshop to purchase additional spiritual books and tapes, etc. During this time the facilitating team meets in a private room downstairs where the meeting is debriefed. Any difficulties that may have arisen are discussed, and reflections on the good points are expressed.

Case Illustration

Catherine M., a 44 year old divorced woman came to the Spirit Life Center 3 years ago extremely depressed. Her parents were divorced at an early age and she had felt abandoned by her father. Growing up she had been repeatedly sexually abused by a family member. She married into an abusive relationship, and her husband abandoned and left her for another woman. There were two children from the marriage, a boy and a girl. Catherine's daughter ran away from home 5 years ago after becoming enmeshed in drugs. Her son, still living with her, has started to exhibit addictive behaviors. He is angry over the decision by the father. She was despairing over losing her daughter.

Before coming to the Spirit Life Center Catherine M. suffered a severe head injury in a car accident which left her cognitively impaired. This deficit affected Catherine's ability to hold down a job, and she was placed on disability. Her former employment was that of a bookeeper. She still does not function well with numbers. Her synapses need to be reconnected. The culmination of all these emotional and physical traumas resulted in a severe clinical depression. Catherine began to attend the ACOK meetings. At first she stayed mute in the back row of the Chapel. This isolation lasted for several weeks. She had become withdrawn from everyone. She withdrew from the other members of Spirit Life Center, and had evidenced little or no faith. She was of Jewish background, but was not practicing her religion.

Initial Intervention

The team facilitators were conscious of Catherine's isolation and need of support. Because of her depression and head injury she had difficulty staying focused. Initially, Catherine began to confide with the Director. Gradually she felt the support and love of the community and began to share her painful story of a myriad of emotional traumas which included sexual, emotional and physical abuse, divorce, desertion of her daughter to drugs, and a fear of losing her son to alcoholism.

Mid-Course Intervention

After several weeks Catherine began to participate in the small groups and to absorb the process of the 12 steps. She started to feel the presence of the Lord, and began to go to other Spirit Life programs. She felt she had a home for the first time, and began to help out in any way she could. As the Director explained the faith to her, she asked whether she could become a member of the RCIA program in her local parish.

Outcomes

There was a lifting of Catherine's depression and she developed a deep joy that culminated in her Baptism into the Catholic faith in her local parish as well as a Baptism of the Holy Spirit. She said that for the first time she felt she was alive. A new sense of enthusiasm entered her life and she began to work in many different programs at the Spirit Life Center.

Long Term Result

At the present time she is a very active member of the Spirit Life Center. She has become a Eucharistic Minister, is the sacristan and coordinates Mass preparations for the weekly Spirit Life Sunday Mass. Since her conversion she also has a deep commitment to her parish. She has become composed and more focused. There is a marked improvement in her physical appearance and emotional demeanor. Unlike others who have established links to Spirit Life Center, she does not fixate on her dependency and truly demonstrates a *newness* of life.

Discussion

It is felt that Catherine has become almost an exemplar of recovery through the 12-Step program and the Spirit Life Community. With the assistance of a spiritual director Catherine is developing a new sense of her own individuality. There has been a re-parenting of Catherine's adult child that is evident in a greater sense of peace and loving responsibility.

References

Jarema, W. (1996). *There's a Hole in My Chest*. New York, NY: Crossroads Publishing.

Linn D., Linn, S.F. and Linn. M. (1993). *Belonging: Bonds of Healing & Recovery*. New York/Mahwah, NJ: Paulist Press.

The Twelve Steps - A Spiritual Journey. (1994). Curtis, WA: RPI Publications Inc.

Woititz, J. (1990). *Adult Children of Alcoholics*. Pompano Beach, FL: Health Communications, Inc.

Key Words

1. *ACOK* - (Adult Child of the King) A program based on the 12-Step concept of A.A. but with innovations that are characteristically unique to the Charismatic prayer meeting and its spiritual format.
2. *Adult Child* - refers to the growth needed for an adult whose *inner child* has suffered trauma during the developmental years.
3. *Baptism of the Holy Spirit* - a deep emotional and spiritual conversion to a personal love of Jesus Christ and his Church which can happen on a personal level or as a group experience.
4. *Charismatic* - a movement which has developed among the Christian Churches, including the Catholic Church, that accentuates the gifts of the Holy Spirit.
5. *Emotionally poor* - those who are unable at a certain time in their development, due to inadequate parenting, addiction, trauma, and conflict, to integrate their emotional, mental and spiritual lives.
6. *Re-parenting* - a process of re-living and re-affirming the emotional child that is within an adult which enables the adult to live a more integrated, productive and spiritually-centered life.
7. *12-Step Program* - a program of spiritual and psychological growth founded on the biblical principles of acceptance, trust in a power greater than oneself, conversion, repentance, and commitment.

Chapter 17

Healing as Restoration of God's Original Intent

Robert T. Sears, S.J., Ph.D.
Loyola University/Gonzaga Hall
6525 N Sheridan Road
Chicago, IL 60626

Practitioner

Robert T. Sears, S.J., Ph.D., received his Doctorate in Spiritual Theology from Fordham University in 1974. He is an Adjunct Professor at the Institute of Pastoral Studies at Loyola University in Chicago. He is also active in doing pastoral counseling, spiritual direction and giving healing retreats.

Training

My dissertation (*Spirit: Divine and Human, the Theology of the Holy Spirit and its Relevance for Evaluating the Data of Psychotherapy* [Fordham, 1974]) treats the theology of the Holy Spirit of Heribert Muhlen (a German Catholic theologian who specialized in the theology of the Holy Spirit) in relation to Freud, Jung and J.L. Moreno's views of therapy. My psychological training was in Psychodrama (group psychotherapy founded by J.L. Moreno), and through study and teaching of C.G. Jung and Theology, Family Systems and Healing, and more recently training in the Restoration Therapy of Serafina Anfuso, Ph.D.

Journey of Integration

My search began during theological studies in Frankfurt, Germany. In seeking the link between therapy and theology I participated in a Psychodrama Congress in Barcelona, Spain and afterwards sought training by Dean Elefthery, M.D. and his wife Doreen. Moreno's group therapy methods were developed by *role-reversing with God* and he led me to see God's and the community's role in healing. At Fordham, I was attracted to Muehlen's theology of the Holy Spirit as *We* in the Trinity, for it grounded the creative community I saw as basic to healing. During this time also, I became involved in the Charismatic Renewal, as well as the revival of the original way of giving the *Spiritual Exercises* of St. Ignatius. During this time, I was introduced to deliverance prayer while working with a person who was both schizophrenic and oppressed by *legions* of demons, and I participated in a workshop on Deliverance given by Francis MacNutt and Fr. Rick Thomas, SJ. I was discovering the practice of healing/deliverance prayer while searching for a theology to undergird it.

I began teaching theology in 1972 in Chicago, where I was introduced by David Augsburger, to Murray Bowen and Family Systems therapy. Bowen correlated well with Muhlen's theology of the Holy Spirit and with Moreno, and I began using healing prayer for the families of persons I was counseling. In teaching "Trinity and Grace," I developed a theology of faith development correlated with the stages of salvation history (see Sears, 1976, 1983) which helped integrate human development with God's way of healing. I joined the Association of Christian Therapists (ACT) in 1981, and became part of a discussion group on inter-generational healing, and another group practicing deliverance prayer. With that help, I could envision healing as cooperating with the interpersonal power of the Holy Spirit, leading each person, as Israel, through suffering and individuation to creative community and love, modeled on Christ's life.

Context

The context of this illustration is a spiritual direction/counseling ministry in a graduate school, the Institute of Pastoral Studies. The directee, whom I will call Lisa, was a student in pastoral counseling who had attended a course I had given which raised issues she wanted to deal with. She came bi-weekly for some 14 sessions, and later brought her husband for a session and referred her sister. I chose her case because of the more extended yet somewhat concentrated time involved in it (I often see people for one or two sessions for intervention prayer to support another therapist, or for an extended spiritual direction time once a month).

Goal

Lisa wanted help with a pervasive depression, and with her relationship with her husband whom she had married two years previously. She had had 6 months counseling before her marriage and again after her marriage, but the depression persisted.

Theory/Theology

God's plan for us is revealed in Genesis and fulfilled through the death/ resurrection of Jesus. We were to form a creative community of self-giving love of male and female, and be fruitful in the image of God's Trinitarian love (see Sears, 1984). God gave us stewardship of creation, and the freedom to make choices that would influence subsequent generations and even the earth (see Sears, 1990, 1994). All this was lost when our first parents distrusted God's love and chose their own way. Alienation from God led to anxiety and shame and disrupted male-female and sibling relationships through blame, control and clinging (the man and the woman), jealousy and hatred (the siblings) and domination rather than harmony with nature. This sinful pattern was handed down in history from parents to children, and is still operative when not corrected by God's redemptive love.

However, God's intention remained and was/is restored through God's interventions in Israel and finally in Jesus' life/death and resurrection. Through Jesus' death on the cross, the Holy Spirit was released to restore our union with God. In the Spirit, God created a new family, symbolized in the relationship of Jesus' mother and the beloved disciple. Thus male-female relationships were healed. Jesus also could command the wind and the sea. He lived a healed stewardship of nature, and has given that authority to us as we cooperate with the Holy Spirit (Sears, 1990).

We recapitulate all the stages of salvation history, culminating in Jesus' death/resurrection/sending of the Spirit. I illustrate five main stages as follows (see Figure 1, taken from Sears, 1983):

1. *Initial faith* is articulated by the Yahwist, an author from David's time (see Genesis 2:3-4 and 12:1-5) who saw the root of evil as distrust in God and disobedience (original sin). Basic trust in God is needed to restore this stage.
2. *Familial faith* focuses on keeping rules and law (the ten commandments) to show faithfulness to God. Sins and blessings of parents are visited on offspring (Exodus 34:6-7; Deuteronomy 5:9-10). Reward or punishment (life or death) is incurred by keeping or breaking the law (see Deuteronomy 30:15-20).
3. *Individuating faith* is God's response when Israel broke the familial covenant and was punished by the Exile. God promised to put his Spirit in their hearts and create a *new covenant* (Jeremiah 31:31-34; Ezekiel 36:24f). Each, from youngest to oldest, would know God and need to choose God (Ezekiel 18). Innocent suffering would open one to a personal encounter with God (Jeremiah and Job).
4. *Communitarian faith* introduces the notion of creating community by suffering for others and forgiving enemies, even non-Jews. It is predicted by Isaiah 53:4-6, but first realized in Jesus whose call to forgive sinners and even Samaritans and Romans brought him the hatred of the Jewish leaders.
5. *Mission faith* expands God's love to all people and all creation. It begins with the resurrection gift of the Spirit at Pentecost, and is expressed by love of all, especially the poor, despite persecution and even martyrdom.

One's living out of the stages is not as clear as they are articulated. One can be in various stages at the same time depending on the area of healing involved. Development is cyclical and the challenges of new stages (like individuating faith) take one back to earlier stages for deeper healing and restoration of the trust God initially intended. Also, breakthroughs in each suc-

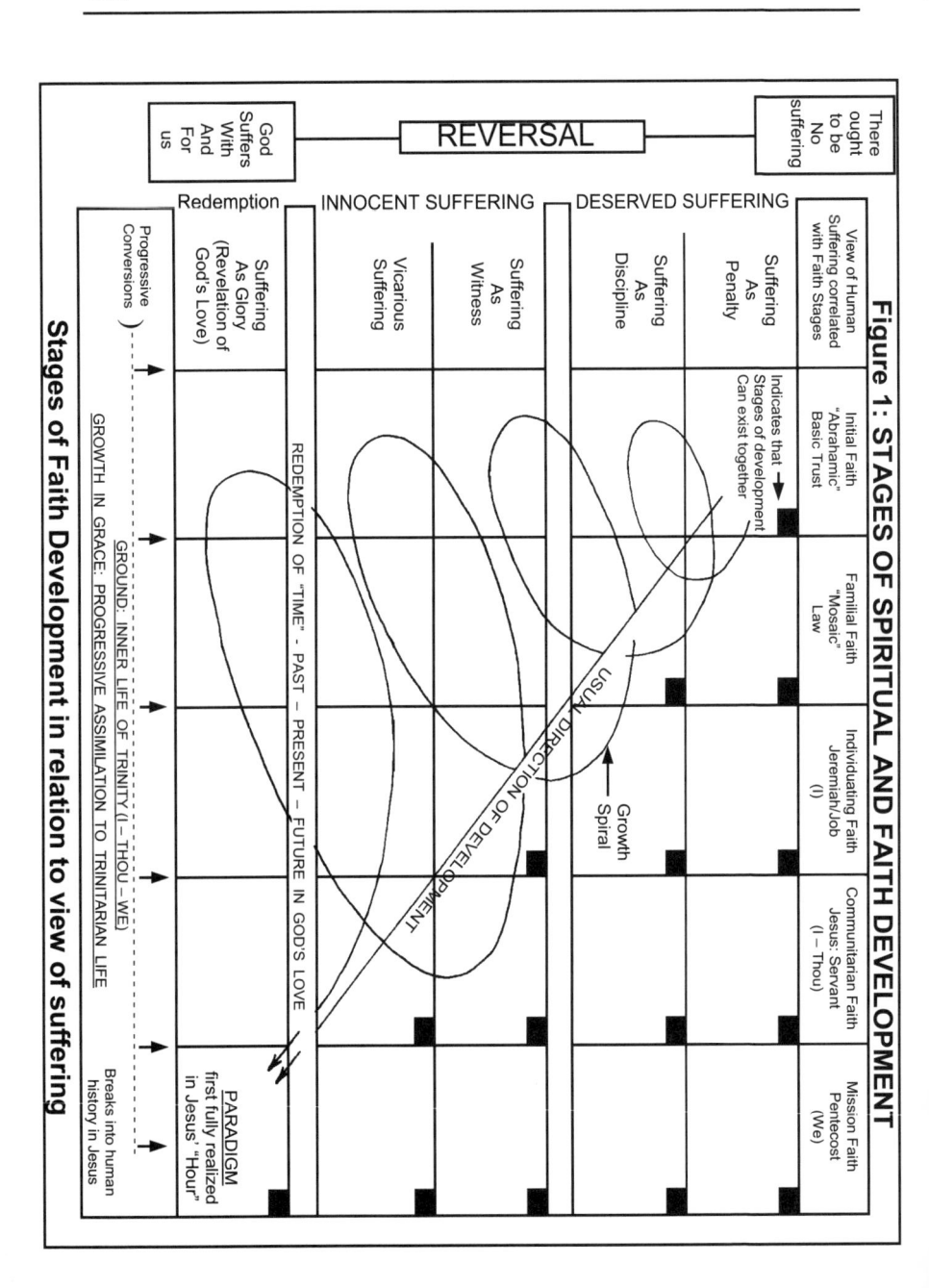

Figure 1: STAGES OF SPIRITUAL AND FAITH DEVELOPMENT

Stages of Faith Development in relation to view of suffering

ceeding stage affect and heal conflicts in the preceding stages. Thus, the final (resurrection) stage confers the power to restore the earliest (trust/ mistrust) stage. It also heals family/ancestors/tradition wounds (second stage), reconnects us immediately to God (third stage) and enables us to bear with others that they might open to healing community (fourth stage). Finally, it heals our relation to our own bodies and all the earth/cosmos (final stage).

The five stages present a map of human development that aids discernment. In dealing with actual issues of a client, I identify nine steps (three groups of three) in opening people to the healing of these stages:

1. *Issue?* (what is the presenting problem? the pain that brings one to therapy?)
2. *Own your feelings around the hurt "wrong"* (anger, sadness, fear, guilt, shame, confusion?)
3. *Who influenced it?* (my mother? her mother? etc. See the context)
4. *Distribute responsibility* (Pray for guidance: what is yours? what others?)
5. *Repent* (change your decision/belief to God's. Ask God to help you find the *basic lie* and your *True Self*, and renounce that *vow* or *basic lie*.
6. *Ask healing* (for the wounds that then surface: the traumas, sins, neglects)
7. *Forgive:* (5 areas: forgive God and ask God's forgiveness, forgive the other and seek their forgiveness, and forgive yourself for your inadequacies.
8. *Intercede* (active care for those that hurt you and ancestors frees you; ask guidance what to do about hurt relationships, ask forgiveness in their name and your own)
9. *Developing grateful mutuality* across generations (goal of healing).

In steps one to three, one identifies the issue and one's feelings around it. In step three, writing a genogram, an illustration of one's family tree, can help one see the influence of parents, ancestry, culture, etc. That opens one to the familial context (my 1st and 2nd stages). Steps four to six focus on personal responsibility and develop individuating faith (my third stage). This gets at what a recent religious therapist has called the *basic lie* (see E. M. Smith, *TheoPhostic* (God's Light) therapy). This core *lie*, which becomes a kind of self-fulfilling *vow*, needs to be changed in light of God's redemptive love in Jesus. Repentance releases the lie and opens to God's truth. Deliverance prayer (for occult or ancestral bondage) may be needed to release the enslaving lie. Releasing the lie opens up the deep pain the lie was covering. One then needs to open to God's healing and ask for it. Steps seven to nine then move one out to bring healing to others, a mark of communitarian and mission faith (my 4th and 5th stages). Having received some healing, one can now forgive the other, God and oneself and open to be forgiven oneself. By forgiving, one sides with God's compassion and gains confidence to intercede for the other that he or she might receive the healing one has experienced. Finally, our awareness of God's healing love can expand to embrace all reality and lead to an ever increasing gratitude - the ultimate sign of healing.

Methodology

The actual method used integrates family systems thought, Jungian insights and faith development in light of God's Word and Scripture. In the initial interview(s) the person's history, especially as related to God, is taken and a genogram constructed. I look for the issue, the blocks that hinder healing (individual and familial), and the positive resources for healing (including the person's spirituality and trust in God, their education and openness to truth). I begin and end a session with prayer, asking for God's enlightenment for the session and praying for healing of the issue(s) discerned.

To illustrate, I will use my own experience of healing. A sense of inadequacy and depression I felt seemed to be rooted in a decision I made very early, perhaps even in the womb, that I *would not be a burden*. I have recently become aware that my decision was a response to my mother's feeling overburdened. To disconnect from my mother's inability to welcome me was an understandable response in the womb, but as an adult I had to accept responsibility for my choice and let it go. Since I was no burden to God, I needed to release the lie that I was a burden. We are responsible for our own responses to painful situations, and cannot blame our parents. Still, I was unable to change the decision by myself. What I did, and what I encourage others to do, was give God permission to change my decision. That is a form of repentance. In letting the decision go, I opened up the pain of my mother not being able to be fully present to me. I then needed to trust that God would make good what my mother could not do - I needed to *seek healing*. Healing came, and is still coming, in a variety of ways: through the intercession of a woman friend, through various healing services, through a therapy training group that I have been part of for several years now. My healing is linked to others' healing. Since my God-image was connected to my parental experience, I had also felt I was a burden to God. That changed as I got a deeper appreciation of Jesus' ministry.

After experiencing that healing I could really *forgive*. Forgiveness is a key to healing as therapists are more and more discovering (see a recent issue of *Family Therapy Networker*, "The Journey to Forgiveness" (Layton, Crenshw & Tangari, Wylie, 1998)). But I have found that we cannot forgive fully until we open ourselves to forgiveness, and to the healing of the wound that hurt us. God needed to begin to heal that mother deprivation before I could let go of the hurt and anger of not receiving the mothering I needed and still need (as we all need parenting). Forgiveness then leads to intercession, as I pray that my mother receive what she could not give to me. And ultimately it leads to gratitude for all aspects of my life, seeing that God brings good even from the hurts.

Case Illustration
Lisa's history

Lisa's maternal grandparents lived with them permanently from the time Lisa was in fourth grade. The three girls were raised very strictly as women by her Hispanic grandmother. They were *very religious* and her sister never dated.

Because of the restrictive home situation, Lisa had been depressed in High School and had difficulty coping. The depression was less pronounced in college where she was freer. After college, several events occurred to bring her again into depression. The boss where she worked became abusive, her boyfriend disclosed he was gay, and her friend and roommate (*Carol*) left her to be with her younger brother whom she had been dating without Lisa's knowledge. Lisa felt deeply betrayed, especially since her family said nothing to her brother about his action. She spent a year in denial and filled her life with work and socializing every night. She sought help from a priest and the church, but with no success, which increased her depression. She then went to a counselor and after a year or so with him quit her job and went to Spain to live with her older married brother. There she read *A Course in Miracles* (for an evaluation of this book see Sears, 1999), devoutly prayed the rosary and spent time in church. She began to work on her own healing. During a visit to Lourdes, she heard the words, *I will send somebody to help you* and the next day in Paris, she met her future husband. While in Spain she became sick and on returning to the USA was diagnosed with hypoglycemia. After a year of trying to resolve her problems herself she became more depressed and returned to counseling. A year and a half later she got engaged and then married. Through counseling the depression lifted enough for her to cope, but a basic anxiety remained even after her marriage. It was after a year and a half of marriage that she entered the graduate program in pastoral counseling at Loyola, and in her second year sought spiritual direction and healing.

Since I had known Lisa from previous course work, I could enter immediately into the background of her issue in her family system. In working

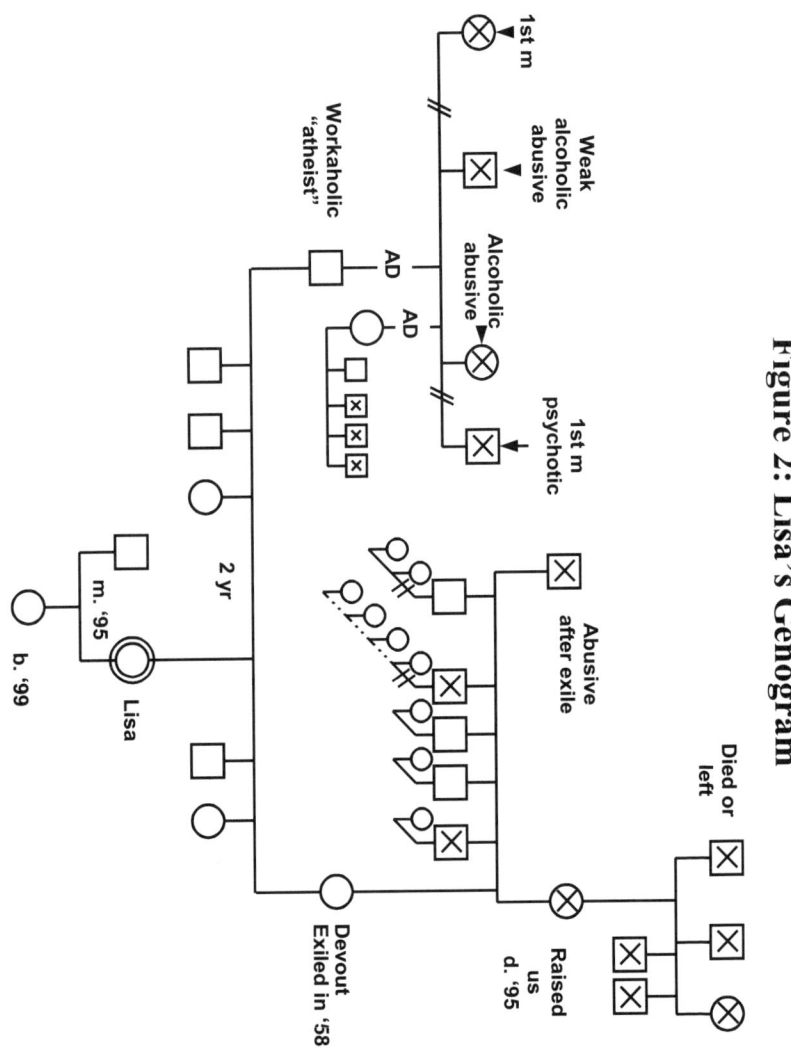

190   A Primer for Christian Healthcare Practice

Figure 2: Lisa's Genogram

with her genogram (see figure 2) she begin to see the pattern of abandonment that was one root of her depression. Lisa's maternal grandmother was brought up by her mother and grandmother. Her biological father either left the family or died. Lisa's mother was exiled from her country when she was twenty, and her mother's father became abusive after the exile.

Another root that appeared was the abuse of power by those in authority. Lisa's father was the older of two adopted children, and knew his stepfather sexually abused his younger sister, who later had a series of failed relationships with men. Both her father and his sister were physically (and sexually?) abused by their adoptive mother who stripped them and beat them as punishment. Lisa's father turned against God and claimed to be an atheist. He coped with life with his mind and was not emotionally available in the family.

I asked Lisa about the part God played in her history. She said that she did not pray to God as much as she used to but was more reflective. She felt abandoned by God and relied more on herself. She claimed to have more *hope* than *faith*, and tended to want to control things. Still, she was open and desirous of having me pray healing prayers.

Processes and Healing Interventions

Having attained the person's background, I look for indications from the directee's experiences and dreams to locate what is surfacing for prayer. In one of the early sessions, Lisa was talking about her father and how he was compulsive and intellectualized everything. She also felt uncomfortable with older men, indeed with men in general. She had a dream in which her husband (Bill) decided it was time for him to grow up. Bill would go to his father and tell him. Bill needed Lisa to come with him, which meant he had to find another wife. Lisa felt she had to go with Bill, but it was not her role. I helped Lisa see her dreams in a Jungian way, as most often representing parts of her own psyche. This empowered her because she saw the dream as a call to individuate from her family– which was not permitted in her family. In the dream, her masculine side (Bill) had to grow up, to reconnect with her father in a mature way and with her feminine side. This moved her toward individuation and to a more mature and equal way of being a wife.

Our prayer, which she found very empowering, addressed both the internal split between her masculine and feminine sides, and the need to reconnect maturely with her father. It went something like this: "Lord, I thank you for your love of Lisa. I ask you to cut her free from the felt neglect of her father so she can recover her own strength. I sever her off from her father's neediness and dominance. Open her to her own masculine strength." Lisa was coming to grips with her own independence and was seeking God's healing (see my steps 4 to 6). She felt empowered when I moved to step 7 and asked her to pray with me for her father that he would be able to forgive his father's incest. "Lord, we stand in for Lisa's father and ask you to release him from the bondage of unforgiveness. Give him the fathering he needs so he can forgive his father and be cut free to find his own strength." Aware of the importance of praying for ancestors (see McAll, 1982; Linn, 1985), I also invited her to pray for the grandfather's healing, asking God to release him from his sin of abuse. We also prayed that her father could forgive his mother's abuse and the wound in his God relationship that resulted from his mother's superficial religiosity. Finally, we prayed that Lisa herself could forgive her father and the *betrayal* of her first boyfriend so she could be free to reunite with her own rejected masculine side. I asked her to express that forgiveness in her own words, and I in turn offered forgiveness in God's name.

There also seemed to be a *vow* involved, a basic *lie* not to trust men. She was able to renounce the vow. I had her write it out in imagination and give it to Jesus on the cross as is done in restoration therapy. We then prayed to God to integrate those masculine qualities in her. "Lord, open Lisa to receive into herself her masculine strength and welcome her wholeness."

In the next session Lisa reported how the doctor she was seeing for hypoglycemia had inquired whether she had ever been suicidal. Though she had not been consciously suicidal, Lisa became aware that she had abandoned her body (abandonment was how her family coped!). This reminded Lisa that a psychic had told her Mom when she was in High School that Lisa would be the person who would most influence her father. For years Lisa had thought, *That's because I am going to die young*, for she could not fathom what else would affect her father in any way. She was getting in touch with her anger that her father did not respond to her. She noted a similar anger against her abusive boss. Recently, she exploded with anger. It seemed that the previous prayer for her father had released the block to her latent anger against men, and had made her aware of a need to heal the split between her body and her *masculine* assertive ego. When we repent (my 4th step) a further need for healing surfaces (my 5th step). This session was concluded with a prayer to integrate her angry side and to reconnect with her body. With her permission, I held Lisa's hands for this prayer, since the wounded child needs touch. "Lord, I thank you for Lisa's anger and her awakened sense of the gift of her body. Help her to welcome her strength and unite her with her body." She experienced a big shift after this, and a dream indicated she was letting her guard down and becoming more receptive toward men in her life.

With growing wholeness, Lisa gained a sense of her own needs and worth. That led her to realize she would want a public apology from the men of her family! Previously she felt very responsible for burdening her family.

Since the family denied negative feelings, she was ashamed to express her needs. Her parents were wealthy, but the children were taught not to ask for things and be spoiled. As she gained self esteem, she noticed in class how she was passed over for 2 days. She felt *invisible*, sad and self-conscious. However, instead of seeking prayer for her own wounded inner child, Lisa asked prayer for her niece (the daughter of her older brother) who was growing bald at 2. As with dreams, I helped her see how *projections* can also indicate parts of oneself that need healing. In praying with her for her niece, I included her own neglected inner child. A later dream showed how things then stood. She was at home by a lake with many children. A man in the dream, who was sitting on a couch and did not want to leave, also felt it was his home. This seemed to indicate a beginning integration of the masculine and her inner children. In another dream, she was in a beautiful pool and had invited a man friend in. Her parents came since it was their home. She was integrating the masculine, but was not yet in her own home.

A later dream indicated a further shift toward fuller inner authority. She found herself alone in a jumping off place. She willingly jumped, though she was scared to death. When she jumped down she passed out. Later she could stand up. It was like an initiation. She was alone. There were a lot of people around but they were not jumping!

In real life, power had been an issue. Her mother had never assumed her power in relation to her father. When Lisa initiated things (like listening to music at night) her caretaker grandmother would barge in and stop her, saying she should be praying. Her dream indicated she was coming into her own inner authority (the individuating faith stage), and we prayed to support God's individual empowerment of her. "Lord, we thank you that you breathe strength into Lisa, and share your own authority with her. Help her to rely ever more on that inner authority that she might be the gift you are empowering her to be."

About this time Lisa became concerned for her older sister who had been brought up in a rigid, fundamentalistic way. Her older sister had met a young Hispanic refugee she had grown to love, but she did not know how to deal with the sexual feelings previously so rigidly repressed. Lisa herself had a strange dream in which she was with a young child (her nephew) and felt herself molesting the child. Lisa's associations with this dream called to mind her Dad's father's incest. She also thought of the desire of 4 or 5 year old children to explore each other's genitals, and of course, her own need to integrate her sexuality. In praying for her sister, we again included Lisa's own need for further integration of her masculine and feminine sides, especially to befriend her own sexual feelings which had been repressed growing up. Integrating one's sexual feelings is often part of individuating faith. Later, I did meet with this sister too, and she experienced an integration and freedom similar to Lisa's. Lisa's healing was having a ripple effect on the family.

Lisa got pregnant toward the end of our time, which led her to bring her husband also for a session. He came from a family where the men were abused and did not stand up to the women. By this time Lisa needed a more equal partnership, and her husband was willing to work on his issues. They since have had their baby and seem to be handling their new life well.

Discussion

This case illustrates most of the dimensions of healing that I discussed: the importance of family systems and healing of ancestors, the stages of development and the different healing needed for different stages, the steps in the healing process and the significance of dreams to indicate what areas are being brought up for healing. It shows the dialectic between praying for one's family and outer relationships and integrating one's inner parts which surface in light of those outer relationships. At the time I dealt with this case, I was only partially trained in *restoration therapy* so I did very little to help her express her emotional states to help her integrate split off parts. Still, those issues and wounded parts did surface and we prayed for their integration.

Let me highlight some of the dynamics that I find operative in this case as in others I have dealt with. First, when Lisa sought spiritual direction and healing, she was open to prayer, but she was also open to addressing her human psychological wounds and acknowledging her part in the process. She did not separate spirituality from human maturation as can happen, and so was empowered by adding prayer to a *higher power* to her counseling experience.

Secondly, Lisa was helped to see a major block when she was introduced to the importance of what Boszormenyi-Nagy (1973) calls *invisible loyalty*. In praying for her father and her grandfather, and extending forgiveness to them, she gained *positive entitlement*. She could begin to be freed from her invisible enmeshment with her father and heal her own inner split between body and spirit, masculine and feminine. She also became freer to connect more deeply with her husband without experiencing disloyalty to her father. Such rejunction with father and mother is essential for a person to be free to commit to anyone else fully (See Sears, 1983).

Thirdly, we find interlocking steps in the healing process. The prayer for her father and her own rejected masculine side led Lisa to recognize she had abandoned her body in the same moralistic way as he had. Her anger with her father (and herself) surfaced and we prayed to integrate it in greater self-assurance. Our prayer for integration with her body opened up her need for family (the mother side?) and her feeling of being overlooked and invisible in her class. In praying for her niece who was two (Erikson's age of autonomy/shame when Lisa's own shyness might have begun) we were strengthening her own sense of self-respect. Her dreams indicated a growing sense of being *home*, that is, in touch with her true self and inner authority. That led her to the sense of needing to *jump*, feeling all alone, with the type of aloneness and *dark night* common to individuating faith. As she experienced her own authority, she was drawn to pray for her sister (the step of intercession) and invite her husband to further autonomy. Both indicate the creative mutuality of *communitarian faith* and show how the healing moved her to restoring the creative mutuality God forever intends.

Finally, prayer was integral to each step and each healing brought her to a deeper view of God's love and desire to heal. Our initial prayer was more petition to separate Lisa from enmeshed *familial* relationships. We gradually moved to a deeper sense of God's involvement in her healing and a more personal trust in God. This growing trust led Lisa to be willing to forgive and intercede for others. She was moved beyond the self-focus typical of *A Course in Miracles* to a more mature interpersonal faith of Christian tradition. We are restored in the image of God's triune love.

Reference Notes:

Anfuso, S. (1994). *Deliverance from Shame*. Roseville CA: Joshua Ministries (5098 Foothills Blvd., Suite 3, Roseville, CA 95678).

_____. (1993). "Spiritual bonding," *Journal of Christian Healing*, 15 *(2&3)*: 28-43.

_____ & Boucher, A. (2000), *Competence and Confidence: Healing Self-Doubt*. Roseville, CA: Joshua Ministries.

Boszormenyi-Nagy, I. And Spark, G.M. (1973). *Invisible Loyalties: Reciprocity in Intergenerational Family Therapy*. New York: Harper and Row.

Bradshaw, J. (1995). *Family Secrets*. New York: Bantam Books. A fine use of family systems with attention to rejunction to one's family.

_____. (1991). *Homecoming*. New York: Bantam Books. Deals with healing the inner child in different ages.

Conn, J. W. (1989). *Spirituality and Personal Maturity*. New York, Paulist Press. A relational view from Kegan.

Crenshw, W. & Tangari, G. (1998). "The Apology," *Family Therapy Networker, 22(6):* 32-37.

Layton, M. (1998). "Ripped Apart," *Family Therapy Networker*, 22(6): 24-31.

Linn, M., Linn, D. and Fabricant, S. (1988). *Healing the Eight Stages of Life*. New York: Paulist Press. Deals with Erickson's stages of growth.

Linn, M., Linn, D. and Fabricant, S. (1985). *Healing the Greatest Hurt*. New York: Paulist Press. Fine on healing across generations.

MacNutt, F. (1995). *Deliverance from Evil Spirits: A Practical Manual.* Grand Rapids, MI; Chosen Books.

McAll, K. (1982). *Healing the Family Tree.* London: Sheldon Press. How prayer for ancestors heals the mentally ill.

Riffel, H. (1987). "Dreams and counseling," *Journal of Christian Healing, 9(2)*: 4-10.

Sears, R. T. (1976). "Trinitarian love as ground of the Church," *Theological Studies, Dec. 1976*, 652-679. This article gives a theological foundation to stages of spiritual development.

_____. (1983). "Healing and family spiritual/emotional Systems," *Journal of Christian Healing, 5(1):* 10-23.

_____. (1984). "Trinitarian love and male-female relationships," *Journal of Christian Healing, 6(1):* 32-39.

_____. (1990). "Resurrection spirituality and healing the earth," *Review for Religious, Mar/Apr.,* 163-177.

_____. (1990). "Jung and Christianity: An interpersonal perspective," *Journal of Christian Healing, 12(2):* 11-19.

_____, with Fritsch. A. (1994). *Earth healing: A resurrection-centered approach.* Livingston, KY: ASPI Publ (Appalacia: Science in the Public Interest, Rt. 5, Box 423, Livingston, KY 40445).

_____. (1999). "A Christian approach to discerning spiritualities." *Journal of Christian Healing, 21(1):* 15-34.

Smith, E. M. (1999). *Beyond Tolerable Recovery: Manual for TheoPhostic Ministry* and the client guide: *Genuine Recovery: Moving beyond tolerable existence into genuine inner healing, renewal and wholeness.* (1996). (Alathia, P.O. Box 489, Campbellsville, KY 42718). Both books and information about training is available from Alathia at 1-(888) 467-3757.

Tyrrell, B. (1982). *Christotherapy II: A New Horizon for Counselors, Spiritual Directors and Seekers of Healing and Growth in Christ.* New York: Paulist Press. A Christ-centered theory of healing spirituality. Follows his *Christotherapy: Healing through Enlightenment.* New York: Seabury, 1975.

Wylie, M.S. (1998). "Secret Lives," *Family Therapy Networker*, 22 (6):38.

Key Words

1. *Restoration Therapy*: A group therapy, developed by Serafina Anfuso (1993, 1994), aimed at restoring initial bonding through prayer and a no JAB (no *J*udgment, *A*dvice or *B*lame) group process using various techniques to release false selves (one's "space suit") and reintegrate one's isolated "inner children."

2. *TheoPhostic Counseling*: A Spirit-guided healing process, developed by

Rev. Ed Smith (1999), that moves from one's pain to core memories and "lies" to praying for God's truth to replace the lies. Experience shows this heals the root of one's pain.

3. *Enslaving lie*: All lies enslave for they are at the root of sin, and sin enslaves. Ultimately, evil spirits have a hold in us only through lies. When the lie is exposed by the truth rooted in Jesus, one is set free (Jn 8:31-4).

4. *Occult bondage*: Negative addictive patterns of experience caused by the influence of evil spirits given entry through wounds, habitual sin, involvement in some form of occult practice (witchcraft, Satanism, spiritualism, etc.) or through ancestral inheritance. Deliverance prayer, or a command in the name of Jesus Christ, is then needed, but always together with healing ministry (MacNutt, 1995).

5. *Positive entitlement*: A term used by Boszormenyi-Nagy to mean the value and merit gained in a relationship by offering due care such as being grateful for gifts received, forgiving, taking steps to help or understand another. Such entitlement frees one to differentiate without disloyalty. (see Ivan Boszormenyi-Nagy & Barbara Krasner, *Between Give and Take: a Clinical Guide to Contextual Therapy* (NY: Brunner-Mazel, 1986).

Chapter 18

Why Have You Forsaken Me?

James J. Wheeler, S.J., M.Div.
St. Joseph's Prayer Center
312 Maple Ave.
Patchogue, NY 11772

Practitioner
James J. Wheeler, S.J., holds a Master of Divinity Degree in Theology, a Licentiate in Philosophy and a Masters Degree in English Literature. He was ordained to the Roman Catholic priesthood in the Society of Jesus in 1968. He has been actively involved in the healing ministry for many years.

Journey of Integration
Though I do not have a degree in psychology, I have read widely in psychology and, of course, spirituality. I underwent a course of studies in preparation for the priesthood and both during that time and since, I have practiced a ministry of spiritual healing and spiritual direction. After I received the Baptism in the Holy Spirit in 1970, I was taught the ministry of inner healing by a Pentecostal woman, Ruth Congdon. I received further instruction in inner healing from others including Agnes Sanford.

After a few years of ministerial practice, I prepared a scriptural course of interior formation in Christ that combined the main themes of the last two thousand years of the history of the Church with the process of inner healing. This course is designed to give the recipient a full spiritual and healing formation. Its name is *The School for Spiritual Growth and Inner Healing*. Over five thousand people have taken this course throughout the world.

In addition, a few years after the first course, there was the need for those who had taken the course in formation, to find and utilize the techniques that the Holy Spirit had taught us in ministry. So we formed the *School of Spiritual Direction*. The implementation of this course on the North American continent resulted in the establishment of thirteen prayer centers in the United States and Mexico.

I have suffered through two periods of depression in my life. One occurred in my adolescent years and early twenties; another occurred recently, in my fifties. After recovery from the last bout of depression, I began to work with other depressed persons by attacking the disease with a combination of spiritual, psychological, and physical means. These practices were

---

* First published in *The Journal of Christian Healing*, Volume 22, Number 1&2, Spring/Summer, 2000, pp. 4-34.

designed to help them through survival in the depressed state and recovery from that state. In that ministry, I completed a book that gives an overall look at helping depressed Christians. The name of the (to be published in Spanish but not yet in English) work is *Why Have You Forsaken Me*. This article is a synopsis of that work as it applied to a particular case.

Context

My ministry is exercised in a setting of spiritual direction, counseling, and healing prayer. I see people (except in emergency or crisis situations) on the average of once a month. Persons with depression generally are seeing a psychiatrist and, in some cases, a therapist. If they work on a particular aspect of their healing or on one of the steps as described below, that month is generally a very productive time. I would like to be able to start depression support groups to help those who struggle to survive the initial and prolonged stage of attempting to endure the horrendous early stages of clinical depression.

Goal

The first therapeutic goal in working with people who are depressed is to give them tools to survive the onset of clinical depression. The survival stage is a time when eighty to one hundred per cent of the person's energies are used to keep the person functioning in their daily life. The next goal is to move the person through the survival stage to the recovery stage. In the recovery stage, the energies of the person turn away from immediate survival and focus on their life tasks.

In the time of recovery, a person who has had a bout of clinical depression should never lose sight of the fact that they have had a bout of depression. They should be well prepared for the symptoms of their own depression, if they should reoccur, so that they might encounter and change them.

Methodology

The methodology that we use has been gleaned from various sources in the professional literature including cognitive therapy, relationship therapy, therapy for past traumatic events, and intergenerational therapy (because depression has been shown to have a familial and ancestral basis). There is a strong emphasis on the techniques of intervention that work for people with depression out of my own experience and the experience of others. Personal interventions should be as simple as possible, attack the depression in its physical, psychological, and spiritual causes and call for the deepest possible relationship with Jesus and with Mary the mother of Jesus, when the person is open to this. This process has been synthesized into fourteen steps in the book, *Why Have You Forsaken Me*. The person suffering from depression relates to these steps in an individual fashion and is encouraged to take what helps and to leave what does not help. These steps are outlined as follows:

I. Jesus suffered depression. Jesus suffered depression on the cross and elsewhere in his life, thus I can come to him with the idea of being understood. Since Jesus is interior to my suffering, I can know or at least believe that he is there with me in my suffering.

II. I can only begin to make my way through this suffering by giving my life entirely over to God without reservation or restriction. When I do this, my depression is not just my problem, it is also God's problem.

III. To survive and to grow, I learn to live in the present moment. I leave the future in God's hand and learn not to get there before I get there. I can prepare for the future but not live in it. Living in the future now is one of the primary causes of depression. Worrying about the future and regretting the past contributes to depression. We must let God bring up the past for healing at the appropriate time: If I bring more trauma into the present before stabilization it may make recovery much more difficult.

IV. I take the medicine that I need. Depression results in a chemical imbalance. Medications can help restore balance. How do I break through the pride of my own self-sufficiency to have the humility to take the medicine that I so drastically need? How do I break through the stigma that society often times places on those who admit that they are depressed and need medication? I participate in the humility of the publican (in the parable of the Pharisee and the Publican, Lk. 18:9-14) by admitting the flaw in my makeup and taking the medicine that I need.

V. Though depression is something I must ultimately work out in solitude before God, I also need others to support me and befriend me during the time of trial. In particular, I need my Veronica, the person who will wipe my face in times of wounding, despondency, and hopelessness. In addition, I need a person who will provide a loving mirror, who believes in me and in my ultimate healing and enables me to see myself as I am. As that person walks with me, I learn to walk with myself as I am. From this arises a realistic hope.

VI. I learn to find the lifeboats *that I need to get through the day.* In each day I must find the particular lifeboats that enable me to survive and persevere. Some of these lifeboats are: physical work, a schedule for the day, doing what I can do and not what I cannot do, exercise, friends, the rosary, Eucharist, understanding consolation and desolation, deliverance and protection, and dealing with insomnia. I also must establish and keep bonds of friendship and not let the heart of love die within me.

VII. I learn to come to live in the mind of the resurrected Christ and to practice resurrection thinking. Resurrection thinking is the ability to come to realistic and positive conclusions at the end of every thought process. This process, which develops gradually, requires that the victim consumed with self pity and blame dies.

VIII. To survive depression, I must embrace a strong belief that God loves me. That belief is founded on the infallible truth that God created me out of his own goodness. That goodness is now accessible to me because Jesus has redeemed me and returned me, by his mercy, into the goodness of my Creator.

IX. Resolution of anger must come and comes only through forgiveness. As I do this, I must also learn how to protect myself, both internally and externally, from abuse.

X. As Jesus tells me continually, "Do not be afraid," I learn to face and walk through my fears with him. I learn to walk through the fear of hell by replying to his unconditional love and learning that he will not betray me nor allow me to betray myself. As I continue to share my fears with him, I learn to place my trust in him and to walk on the water with Jesus and with Peter.

XI. When I come to accept the realities of my life, including the depression I am working through, I open the door to deeper resources of inner peace and understanding myself. In understanding myself and the triggers of depression, I learn not to let judgment of others, self judgment, and oppression into my life. I accept my life and work through depression one day at a time.

XII. Learning to walk through darkness. I learn that the Lord works through darkness and desolation as well as through light and consolation. I learn to walk by faith and not by sight. When I persevere in faith and in the darkness, I begin to find the presence of the Father in my life.

XIII. The power of restoration. Our God is a God of restoration. I must learn to rely on him to protect, sustain, and deliver me as I enter the darkness of depression and then to restore me. I do this in prayer to him who knew me and loved me before the foundation of the world.

When I am walking in survival, I ask the Lord to heal me to maintain the powers of mind, will and mobility that seem to be in danger. As I enter recovery I begin to ask Jesus for the powers of mind, will and mobility that I have lost or found to be inactive during the depression. In the power of restoration these powers can be restored to me in active life. I also ask for the restoration of the relationships that can be accomplished without damage to me.

XIV. Resurrection: in the time of recovery, I experience the fullness of growth in the resurrection of Jesus. The fullness of the resurrection is the helping of others through their depression. No suffering goes unused.

Jim's Story and Karen's Story
Step I: In identifying with Jesus, who suffered depression himself,
   I find that I am not alone

During my first experience with depression, I remember looking for someone with whom I could identify. The only people that came to mind were the poor people of Auschwitz. It seemed that they were the ones who felt the way I felt. Only they would understand the sense of hopelessness and total endless darkness afflicting my spirit day by day. I could make no claim to suffering the persecution they underwent. However, the continuous inner negativity, the revolt of the mind that persecuted the spirit with endless hostility, gave me an inner picture of what they suffered interiorly and exteriorly. I gave no pretense that my suffering equaled their suffering, but in my desperation for someone to identify with, these people crossed my mind. They would understand and commiserate with my endless bath of persecution. They might be the ones to show me the way to hope in the midst of inner darkness. At the time they were a source of comfort. There were people in this world who could understand.

Those days are long gone from my life, but permitted me to understand a woman who came to me for help. I will call this woman Karen (not her real name). Karen was suffering a relentless inner darkness and was experiencing continuous negativity which followed her spirit like the continuous snap of a sharp and biting whip. Her face showed signs of continuous insomnia. Karen's recovery was not to be dramatic and complete. She had to work for some time before the glimmer of recovery would touch her troubled spirit.

It Takes Time: I have chosen Karen's story because it is not a case in which sudden and miraculous healing takes place. Her story has to do with the healing of her entire life and discovery that the only way to resurrection was through accepting the cross that was present in her life. Her healing required time, in which she came to accept the cross of depression. This played an essential part in her survival and eventual recovery.

In my own healing, the passage from survival to recovery would take time. During that time, I found that the biggest contributors to my survival were people who spent time with me without judging me and who supported me without demanding I be someone who looked or felt better than I actually did.

For Karen, the thing that was so helpful was the fact that I had been through what she was suffering. Because of my experience with my own depression, I could understand what she was going through and validate her suffering. For Karen and many with depression, the fear exists that they are totally insane or at least out of their minds. For another to validate their feelings and say that this is part of a specific disease enables them to put boundaries on that fear and the negativity of their imagination.

To know that another person accepted their feelings without rejection or judgment, can affirm that they have a specific disease and are not insane. The minister of healing can, in no way, be the savior of another person, but their openness to hear the fear and anxiety of the afflicted one, can open the door for the client to the belief that God is with them. This is a form of divine mediation in which the person who is suffering can begin to believe that Jesus is really there for them and receives their suffering and pain.

Karen: Perhaps one of the reasons people fall into depression is that their heart dies. They are unable to find the way to love and be loved in life. This is a difficulty for all of us, the primary challenge of life and of Jesus who found the way to love not only his enemies but his friends. The life of happiness and real joy is to find the way, with Jesus, to love both friends and enemies.

This was a real difficulty in Karen's life. It became apparent that from the very beginning Karen suffered a great deal of deprivation in some of her fundamental relationships. Karen never really bonded with her now deceased father. Her memories of her mother consisted of verbal abuse and threats of physical abuse, and an irrational anger or hatred which made Karen fearful. Karen's mother had been divorced from her husband, a person who seemed incapable of giving real love. In these key relationships a death had occurred in Karen's heart, a death which kept depression alive.

Karen had not curled up inside herself and let herself die. Despite these extraordinary deprivations in her own life, and the chronic tiredness due to insomnia, she still sustained several friendships. These friends provided constant support in her life. She prayed with them and they helped each other through the difficulties. She also belonged to a prayer community where she used her spiritual gifts to help others. Through her own courage and persistence, she avoided one of the pitfalls that can make depression more terrible and more chronic, isolation and the fear of relationships. Karen was not isolated and continually afraid of relationships. Yet the fundamental deprivations, in her parental and married life, cast a shadow over her existence.

The Role of the Imagination: In my own inner healing, imagination played a major role. First, I would ask and imagine Jesus and Mary coming into those parts of my past where I had sustained wounds for many years. This proved to be a deep source of healing. A second practice of entering into those places of the life of Jesus where his experience and my experience were similar always provided me with a source of healing and identification. However, many of these experiences did not help me in my time of depression. At times I was reluctant to use them with Karen. However, because of her alienation, I decided to see if Karen could ask Jesus to come into those painful memories. She resisted, but like a soldier, she worked her way through, relating her experiences to Jesus' experiences in scripture. I wondered if this was helpful. Karen told me later that they were helpful.

Karen had to learn what is taught in most therapy: how to protect herself from being a constant victim. Against abusive and non-responsive parents, she (and her little child) had to find the boundaries that were necessary to protect her from abuse and deprivation. She had to find out that she was not guilty of that lack of love and severe accusations that had been poured upon her. But, besides being safe and secure, Karen had to learn something else.

Jesus has told us to love our enemies. Jesus allowed himself to be exposed to their severe abuse and torture only once. At other times he was safe and secure from the instruments of hate.

But Jesus, through the forgiveness and love of his enemies, taught us something very crucial. Though we seek safety and security from our enemies, the secret to the fullness of heart and the wholeness of the complete heart of love is to find the way to love them.

Jesus would not let his own heart die by not loving those who had harmed him. He would not allow their hate to steal from him the power of love. He still continued to forgive them and love them.

Asking Jesus into the painful memories allowed Karen to begin to open up a prayerful relationship with her mother, father, and husband from whom she had been alienated. Once she had established sufficient boundaries between herself and these others, she was free to forgive and free to open her heart in love towards them. The part of her heart that died began to live again. But, if she were to recover, she also had to learn to avoid the deprivation that happens when love collapses and cannot recover. It is in this place of unlove that her heart slowly died when she turned her love off from those who hurt her. Yet *with* Jesus and *in* his wounded heart she learned about the power of forgiveness and the healing power of being joined with him in a love for others that *refuses to die*. In her prayer for her *persecutors* she received healing of the dead part of her heart and was able to begin to open her heart to the healing love of Jesus in those broken relationships.

Because of difficulties in her relationships with her mother, her father and her husband, Karen was unable to take steps towards real reconciliation. Continuous prayer enabled God to heal, at least in part, the deprivation experienced in these relationships, one of the sources of the depression.

Karen and Step I: Karen had difficulty with regard to Step I. She did not see Jesus' suffering on the cross as something she could fully identify with. For her, Jesus suffered only for a short time while she suffered for a number of years. How could Jesus appreciate her suffering over a long period of time when he, though enduring horrendous tribulation, had seen it end in a few hours?

To appreciate any of the mysteries of the life of Christ, especially the mystery of the passion of Jesus, the mind must suspend its objective judgment. The full mystery of Christ can be revealed only to a mind that is able to see that mystery by the power of grace.

In my case the inner revelation of the suffering of Christ was key in my recovery. I also realized that Jesus' suffering had only been for a short time. However, when I let go of that judgment, I realized that Jesus' suffering had such intensity and extended to all time and to the sin and suffering of all mankind. Then I stood in awe before this incredible mystery.

In the midst of my own depression a deeper realization appeared in my mind. After his death and resurrection Jesus could not personally suffer in his own body and in himself. But he could suffer in the way a mother or father in their love for their child in pain suffers. The mother or father does not suffer in their own body, but when they see their children suffer, they, too, suffer in their spirit. Jesus no longer suffers in his own body, but he does dwell within us. He suffers the consequences of our sin and is closely related to our own suffering. Jesus, who is more intimate to us than we are to ourselves, who is more intimate to our suffering than even we are, suffers in us and with us.

That Jesus' personal suffering ended is a reality. But the fact that he endures our suffering and in some deeply mysterious way suffers in my suffering and suffers in the suffering of all on this earth for all time, overwhelmed me. I could now come to know that he, who perhaps had suffered more deeply than me was now deeply interior to my suffering. He was my brother in the midst of my suffering. He knew what my suffering was. He the Lord of us all, who had in some sense suffered all of our suffering by becoming Lord, he was the one who was holding me in his hands in the midst of my suffering. This realization overwhelmed my heart and allowed me to soften and to surrender to his embrace in the midst of my own terrible suffering. I was no longer standing apart from him, judging his suffering and its limitations. I could embrace him now as someone who fully understood my suffering. I knew that he who is compassion itself, had more empathy for my suffering than I did. He had died on the cross for my suffering and I now knew what that meant.

Karen's Gift of Understanding: Karen had difficulty identifying with Jesus the way I had, but in her own way, she pursued the first step. She found her way into one of the great secrets of the spiritual life, namely that God is not only found in light or consolation, but God is also found in darkness and desolation. In enduring her tiredness and wandering years in the desert, she came to the intuition, that, in the midst of the night and the deep desert, God is found. When I asked her how she was able to endure all that she endured, she remarked, "Well, I believe that Jesus has been with me. Out of that belief there has come the powerful sense that he is always there. No matter how bad the depression and how much I am suffering, I know that he has always been there." In reality she jumped from the first step of the program to the twelfth step, the step of the dark night of St. John of the Cross, where God is discovered in the dark night in the soul.

In this mystical journey, understanding of the movement from a tangible experience of God to a sense that God is not here has to be dealt with. Then, that which first appears as abandonment becomes the deepest gift of the soul. For one discovers God, not in an emotional manner, such as the attachment to God's consolation, as in the early stages of the spiritual life, but in surrender to God. Instead of demanding that God be someone I use for my spiritual pleasure, I, like Jesus, relate to God in the darkness of the desert, in the midst of intense suffering. When I slowly begin to perceive that God is there in the deepest part of my soul, and in the depth of my tribulation, then I can realize that God lives in the center of my suffering.

Here the miracle of the inner life occurs. When I accept this opaque but very real experience, I am prepared to accept God into the deeper parts of my soul. God can enter the secret part of me that is unseen by anyone, the place in which my inner will, inner heart and inner mind exist. In this secret part of me, God lives, hidden, unknown except to me who deeply know of God's presence and enduring companionship.

Karen had reached and touched the inner part of God's relationship to her. Instead of resenting God's non-appearance in her emotions and moods, she found God at the place where her cross and God's cross touch in the center of her being. Because she was still suffering greatly, she did not fully appreciate the gift she received, but I could see it from the beginning. There was an inner beauty, a luminosity in her that was evident from the very beginning. When she told me about the gift she received, the reason for her inner light began to appear.

Step II: Giving one's life entirely over to God
In the presence of Jesus Karen began to understand that she could have a relationship with the Father. This is one gift that can appear in depression.

To begin the journey through the nightmare of depression, one can use psychological means and medication. But this will not begin to solve the terrifying alienation those with depression experience. The direct counter measure in the spiritual realm that can begin to ground someone in the battle with depression is something I learned from *Homes for Growth* in Winnipeg, Canada. (*Homes for Growth* is a place where people go for recovery from trauma and depression. They stress a deep surrender to God and a deep reflection on who we are as a way to recovery.) In order to fight this battle, Jean Wilmot, the leader of the *Homes for Growth*, said that we had to put our whole life into the hands of God. We had to give ourselves entirely over to God so that the battle, which really could not be fought alone, could now be taken on as a joint venture.

After I gave my life over to God, the depression was not only my problem, but was God's as well. This surrender of myself completely to God had a strong effect on me. I no longer felt I was walking on sand, but now was on solid ground despite the turmoil, the darkness, and the fear I still had. Somewhere at the bottom of my spirit I was walking on solid ground even though other parts of me were continually walking a stumbling, broken gait. This step was the beginning of a mutual journey with God our Creator to understand what happened to me. It was to know, as I continued the process of total surrender, that even though I continued to be depressed, God the Father was walking with me, as he walked with Jesus through the deep temptations of the desert.

This type of total surrender, like the total *fiat* of Jesus on the cross, seemed key in my relationship with the Father. In Karen's case, she had to make this total surrender to God again and again. In this process, she too became more grounded, felt as if she was walking with Jesus, and, in the deep part of her being, felt a strong connection to Jesus and the Father. In the process of surrender, Karen began to experience something that I had also experienced.

Though I always had a faith relationship to the Father, the process of continual surrender led me closer and closer to the Father, until, after several years, a companionship with him was fostered. The Father was no longer distant, but somehow walking right beside me. The relationship with the Father that would heal the core of my being and lead me, by the surrender of mind and heart and will, into the very center of divine love, fostered the giving over of each day to the Father.

And so it was with Karen. In the patient endurance of this deep trial, in the continual surrender again and again, she developed an intimacy with the Father. By walking through her suffering with God, Karen began to understand that she did not have to remain in a position of anger and resentment. Through the power of forgiveness and love, she could trust her deep instinct to stay with God through the carrying of her cross. Through the acceptance of that terrible journey, Karen, like Jesus and Mary before her, began to deepen her companionship with the Father.

The practice of Centering Prayer was a continual help for Karen. (Centering prayer is a form of contemplative prayer described by Fr. M. Basil Pennington, OCSO in *Centering Prayer: Renewing an Ancient Christian Prayer*

Form and also developed by Abbot Thomas Keating in many of his books, see *Open Mind Open Heart: The Contemplative Dimension of the Gospel.*) In this kind of prayer one bypasses the thinking processes of the rational mind by turning one's mind to the inner presence of God. Centering prayer enabled Karen to detach, to some extent, from the darkness and pain in her life. She was able to focus her mind simply on God and to experience some relief from the depression and her continuous exhaustion. In addition, prayer seemed to give her strength and the ability to detach even when she was not actively praying. At times she would be in such pain that she really could not bear it. At those times she would prostrate herself before the crucifix.

We had to deal with some negative effects of centering prayer. This prayer tended to make her spacey at times. It provided an escape from the difficult work of dealing with her deprivation and negative emotions that fostered it. At times she, because of her suffering, was susceptible to running away from the work she needed to do. We attempted to compensate by using focusing prayer. (Focusing prayer is a technique discovered by Maurice Gendlin. It was further developed in a Christian way by Ed McMahon and Peter Campbell in *Bio-Spirituality: Focusing as a Way to Grow.*) This is a technique which emphasized the feelings in her body and the imaginative prayer which brought about a more concrete emphasis on the events of her life.

Step III: Living in the present moment
One of the constant themes of Christian spirituality is living in the present moment. To stay focused on what is presently in front of me is a good therapeutic device and brings about better productivity in life. It is also a way in which we can live constantly in the presence of God. By offering each moment to God and living in that moment, we come slowly into God's presence as we do our daily work and interrelate with others. After a time one becomes aware that God is there in all we do, even if we feel desolation or the lack of God's presence in our formal prayer.

Living in the present moment brought me into a concrete sense of God's ever abiding presence in my life through five years of terrible desolation. For those with depression, the power to live in the present moment brings other benefits. To live in the present moment is to leave the future in God's hands. That brings a tremendous sense of relief. *I live in the present, let God take care of the future. Do not get there before you get there. Prepare for the future, do not live in the future.*

To live by the maxims italicized above is to remain in the present. To live in the energy of the now moment and survive in that moment, a new hope is born in the person, a hope that is founded on the rock of the present.

Those with depression are constantly concocting negative or catastrophic visions of the future. This tendency to live in the future is constantly draining on the personality, produces continuous anxiety and makes the person enter into deep fatalism, with the tendency to give up hope and believe that life will end in something horrendous. The worst thing that one can do is give up hope.

For Karen, knowing how to live in the present moment was a great gift. She did not have to bear the burden of past suffering in the present, or carry the burden of her depression into an endless future. She could live through each moment, survive each moment. A future whose negativity or catastrophic elements were always before her was unlivable. For Karen removing the obsession with the future by living in the present was a necessary part of survival and a part of living. To focus on an endless future filled with depression was an unbearable predicament. To live one day at a time was a tolerable way of dealing with her reality.

In Karen's life the concentration on living in the present moment was vital to her ability to survive and keep going on. In times of financial crisis she was thrown out of the present. Her trust in God predominated and she returned to living in the present. The present moment was a rock she could grasp allowing her to survive the present storms and keep the future from killing her.

Step IV: Medication

Accepting medication can be difficult when one first discovers the terrible vicissitudes of clinical depression. It was for me. To me, needing to take medication was to admit that I was not *normal*, that I suffered from mental illness (no matter how common that illness). To let go of my pride and say that I was not like other people was difficult, something like admitting leprosy must have been in times past. I felt banished into a condition that made me less than a regular human being. This acceptance strikes at the very heart of societal shame and involves such a breakdown of normal human pride, that it was almost impossible to do. I could only do it when the pain became so bad that I knew medication was the only way out.

Even then I discovered that I was not on the right medication. I was overwhelmed by anxiety and intellectual scruples. Finally, I changed psychiatrists and medication. I was still over-medicated. Terminating the medication, I was still left with the fear of medication. It took me four years to find a small dose of the right medication that would provide me with the final step.

Karen had even more difficulty with medication. We advise those with depression to take medication if they need to. Karen had tried many medications - about a dozen in all. With each one she had severe side effects and was not able to continue. Thus, for three years, she had to battle insomnia and other symptoms without the serotonin her body needed. A series of traumatic events led to her being able to stay on a medication. Even then, the amount was limited by a side effect - severe dry mouth - making her unable to swallow. She was able to take some medication that helped her to sleep. She was able to work full time, but struggled with fatigue and sleep deprivation. The medication helped to some degree, but it did not end her problem.

Step V: Though I must face the depression alone, I need the support of friends to get me through it

In Jesus' battle with the depression of Gethsemane and Calvary, he met a remarkable woman along the way of the cross. Veronica* knew she could not take the cross away from Jesus. She knew that the terrible thing happening to him was inevitable. She could not save or rescue him. She could show a touch of love and demonstrate she was with him, understood his suffering, and sensed the deep injustice taking place. As Jesus carried his cross and approached Veronica, his face was covered with blood because of the crown of thorns and the blows he had received. Veronica did something that would be recognized for its courage and its deep love. Veronica wiped Jesus' face tenderly and lovingly with her veil.

There were many along the way who were unable to rescue Jesus. They were unable to stop the terrible thing that was happening, but they were there. They showed their love: the weeping women, Simon of Cyrene who helped Jesus carry the cross, Mary, Susannah and Mary, the Mother of Jesus with John the beloved disciple. They were all representatives of the Father who could not save Jesus either, but who sent those to love him and provide the support, compassion, and strength that he needed to make it through his death and resurrection.

In my own battle with depression, I needed the Veronicas. I knew that no one but Jesus could save me and get me through. None could rescue me, but the Veronica's were there for me, staying for an hour or two, taking me to lunch, taking a walk with me, showing me that they cared. These were the people, who by the gentle caress of their friendship, enabled me to go on one day at a time. The people who stayed away could not help me. The people who tried to save me or tell me to get better could not help me. Only those who cared by showing they were there with me when I was down and befriended me in my desperate moments, were the ones who saw me through.

Karen had several people who really loved her with the genuine friendship that supports a person through good times and bad. These people talked with her, met with her, gave her words of knowledge, and were there when times were strained and difficult. Karen was a spiritually gifted person and

---

* The legend of Veronica wiping the face of Jesus is told in the fifth station of the Christian devotion called *The Stations of the Cross.*

was able to use her gifts to help others. Her gifts of prophecy and word of knowledge were very helpful to many (see I Cor. 12 for St. Paul's discussion of the gifts of the Holy Spirit). She continued to raise her daughter. Despite the terrible odds of fatigue and depression, she was able to be there for others. This allowed her to avoid the trap of always being cared for and never being able to care, a difficulty that could result in a sense of continual psychological debt. *Doing what you can do,* a motto I learned from handicapped people in Canada, helps someone in depression avoid this kind of debt.

The legend of Veronica holds a second gift. The legend says that Jesus, after the touching consolation of having his bloodied face wiped, left the imprint of his face on the veil. The power of the story is that Jesus was truly seen, his suffering truly known by Veronica. She provided a loving mirror for him to see himself. She saw him as he was. She saw the immense suffering and disfigured face, yet did not turn from him in horror or disgust, but reflected her love back to him in the gesture of the veil she offered to cleanse his face.

In each of my depressions there has been someone who was a loving mirror, someone who loved me in a way that allowed my suffering to be seen, and returned that vision of what sometimes was torture, anxiety or borderline despair. The return of the vision was with compassion and love. It truly enabled me to survive, knowing that despite everything, I was still understood and loved by another.

Another quality or grace of Veronica was that she, by her gesture and her love showed that she believed in Jesus. I once asked another with depression what was the thing that enabled her to recover. Her response was that her therapist believed in her. I know the great gift of those who, in my six years of depression, continued to believe in me. They mirrored Christ's belief in me and they showed me by their love, the precious gift in Veronica's veil. It enabled me, once I had recovered, to be a loving mirror and to give the gift of faith, the faith of Jesus to so many others with depression. This included Karen.

Step VI: Lifeboats: The things that get you from one moment
    to the next moment or one day to the next

In the list of lifeboats there are many things that helped Karen make her way through depression. Centering prayer, continually supportive friends, an inner knowledge of how much stress she could take and when to rest and physically exercise, were all things that helped her to survive over seven years of depression. A combination of five things made a significant difference in her progress: *community, deliverance prayer, intergenerational healing Mass, daily Mass & Eucharist and adoration of the Blessed Sacrament.*

1) Community—Karen lived in a Christian community that was very supportive. This was one factor that enabled her to survive. The community was in constant contact with her and she developed several significant friends in the community. This continuous support was a very crucial factor to help her through the deep purgatory in which she found herself. Within community, the charismatic gifts of the Holy Spirit were present, in particular, the word of knowledge. The word of knowledge is a gift of the Holy Spirit that leads the minister of healing to areas significant to the person's recovery. In Karen's case, a member of her community received a word of knowledge about her maternal grandmother while praying with Karen. It seemed that the grandmother had been involved in occult practices and had placed several curses upon her family. These curses had an effect on Karen. She needed to be delivered.

2) Deliverance—Based on the word of knowledge, I confirmed that the maternal grandmother had placed these curses on Karen's family. I brought the Blessed Sacrament into the room. She knelt and I blessed her three times with the sacrament. She in turn blessed herself, renounced the curses of her grandmother and the negative or evil part of the relationship through which they had been channeled.

3) Intergenerational Healing Mass—Within a short period of time, we had an intergenerational Mass. In this Mass we asked forgiveness not only for our own sins but for the sins of our ancestors. Included in this Mass is a deliverance prayer said at the Our Father. This plus the original deliverance prayer had a remarkable effect on Karen. From that time on, the spirits of torment, terror and torture which had been a constant part of her life were removed. She was still bothered by depression but these spirits, which had been a constant source of stress and distress, were gone from her life.

4) Daily Mass & Eucharist—Daily participation in the Eucharist is a time of consolation, an oasis of peace, that is essential for surviving depression. Another of my clients who was hospitalized with a manic depressive episode found the Eucharist and the intimate relationship with Jesus were the essential lifeboats that kept her on the track in her survival and recovery.

The beautiful ritual movements in the Mass: Offertory, Consecration, Our Father, and Communion, along with the reading of the Word of Scripture, are sources of grace and provide a door to the Divine Presence that are not felt anywhere else. For those in depression, who are trying to survive desperately in the beginning, the presence of Jesus, so tangible and physical in the Mass and Eucharist, is a window to the unseen light of God, and a touching apparition of the Divine Presence that is found nowhere else in life. In terrible moments of despair and deep anxiety, where God seems to have disappeared, Jesus can suddenly return in the sacrament of the Eucharist. For those in depression, as for all the other refugees working their way through various forms of hopelessness, the Eucharist is the unique form of God's redemptive justice to those who feel abandoned by God and man. In the reception of the Body and Blood of Jesus in the Eucharist, the depressed person, feeling deserted by God and man, is singularly aware that the presence of the Body and Blood of Christ in his or her body is the tangible and material confirmation that he or she has not been deserted.

In Karen's case receiving the Eucharist had been a life long devotion. In her pursuit of God even before her battle with depression, she had found that the Eucharist was a lifeline. It was her way of reaching God and of touching the only person who gave reality its essential meaning—Jesus. In the days of depression, listening to the Word proclaimed to her, offering to God the reality of her life, becoming aware of God's divine presence at the everyday miracle of the consecration and receiving God into her body and spirit, created a necessary moment of tranquility in a life that always bordered closely on desperation.

Karen needed prayer to be a central part of her life. As she began her recovery and found enough energy to work a full-time job, her prayer time at night was diminished. She had to care of her daughter, prepare herself for the morning, and retire early. In these circumstances the Eucharist became the focus of her personal prayer. In the Eucharist she found the support for her fragile life. Eucharist continually helped her to get through each day and gave her courage to face the daily battle with insomnia.

5) Adoration of the Blessed Sacrament—I have found two things to be of great significance in the spectrum of Christian practice: praying the rosary and adoration of the Blessed Sacrament. In sitting or kneeling before the Blessed Sacrament, the distressed person often finds an oasis of peace. The conflict and turbulence of depression or other diseases can be muted considerably by time spent in the presence of Jesus in the Blessed Sacrament. In his presence, peace of mind can be revived; one has a sense that God is there and concerned and insights are found to help carry on in times of great difficulty. Decisions that need to be made become clear and the areas of the personality that need to be strengthened and purified are found. The presence of Jesus, often so tangibly felt in the Blessed Sacrament, is the sign to all who suffer, including those with depression, of God's care and concern in the midst of their personal passion.

Karen spent two hours a week in front of the Blessed Sacrament. There she would find peace and tranquility that were absent from her ordinary life. Using adoration and centering prayer, she reached a place of inward peace.

This was a great blessing, telling her of the place where she and God were one and where she could, for an hour or so, be free of fatigue and suffering so characteristic of her life. She described this time as a time of inner peace that made her relationship with Jesus more visible and tangible. She could, in those moments, "fill herself with God," "find a solution to her problems," and "become real in her relationship to Jesus." In addition, although suffering from continuous insomnia and (to this day) fatigue, before the Blessed Sacrament, Karen found a deep rest for body and spirit.

Step VII: Resurrection Thinking

One woman suffering with depression made a remarkable statement that was the best attempt I know of to define depression. She said that depression is a *revolt of the mind*. When you are depressed, the mind seems to go into a negative space. It tends to see things with a perpetual negative inclination. Catastrophes are about to happen momentarily. Negative roadblocks seem to occur everywhere. The mind enters into a perpetual prophetic state of doom and gloom. Everyone around the person with depression is suspected of negative judgments about that person's work, life, and personhood. This negative bombardment, at least in the beginning, is relentless.

I tried the approaches of cognitive therapy and found them somewhat helpful. However, I found the rational types of thinking required of me to be impossible. My mind had great difficulty even thinking about how to survive and was unable to do procedures required in cognitive therapy. Later I realized that the approaches of cognitive therapy involved the therapist's continual interaction with the client, an interaction that was impossible for me.

Rather than abandon this approach, the Lord intervened. I received inspiration from the Holy Spirit called *Resurrection Thinking*. In the beginning that meant simply drawing on the resurrected power of Jesus Christ in his Spirit and thinking as positively as I could in every circumstance. My mind was so negative at that point, that the extreme of continuous positive thinking, in the resurrected mind of Jesus, rather than cause distortion, served simply to balance thinking. This give me the power to do things that otherwise seemed impossible. I continued in this stage for some time but realized over time that this approach needed modification. If allowed to go on perpetually, it might result in fanciful, manic or *Mary Poppins* thinking. I realized that resurrection thinking involved *realistic thinking as well as positive thinking*, in other words, thinking that was *realistically positive.*

If, in my depression, Aunt Tillie's coming was viewed as a disaster, then I certainly could prophesy:

1) that she would drive me up the proverbial wall, and
2) that her judgments were ones that I would take into myself and let them tear me apart.

If I thought this way, Aunt Tillie might be the person to push me into a continuous state of depression. If I could leave Aunt Tillie in the hands of God and live in the now moment, then the draining and anxiety-ridden perspective of Aunt Tillie's coming might be temporarily eclipsed. I could gain the energy needed for this encounter. That may be all I could do.

After a while, the mind can change from its doomsday mentality. Aunt Tillie's coming might be a time to practice detachment and learn how to set boundaries with intrusive and codependent harridans who continue to harass. I could greet Aunt Tillie's judgmental comments with silence; and then, I would ask Jesus for the power to reply without playing into her game. I could ask Mary, the Mother of Jesus, for the gift to get around the road block created by Aunt Tillie's comments. I could also ask God for the grace not to take in the sinfulness of Aunt Tillie's negative judgments, rejections, and gossip. In other words, I can, by entering into the resurrected mind of Jesus, begin to change the perspective I have in mind and begin to transform a negative event into a very positive event.

Karen often practiced positive thinking. This enabled her to deal with reality with the mind of the resurrected Christ and enabled her to be free of negative and catastrophic thinking that brings the mind and the spirit down. Even though life was difficult, Karen managed to maintain a positive attitude. This attitude, the changing of the mind by the grace of hope, brought her the gift of survival.

Step VIII: To believe that God loves me and that God has created me out of God's goodness

In my own staggering through the wasteland of depression, I found that the greatest ally I had was the gift of faith. As I traversed the mine fields of depression and anxiety, I found the only thing to hold onto was Jesus, my Lord and my God. Faith in him would remain in the darkness and the light, through the anxiety and the deep dives into the varied forms of hopelessness that depression offers. He, through faith, would remain the rock that never failed me. I often wondered if I was living in the same faith that my ancestors in Ireland did who had to make it through so much inward and outward famine, war, and depression.

After a time I had to find a way to fire into me this gift of faith. In the midst of waves of negativity I held fast to the fact that God had created me out of God's goodness. Of course, we lost that connection by our sinfulness. Jesus, through his life, death and resurrection and the confession of our sins, redeems us. He, by the mercy of God returned to us the relationship to the Father that was lost in the Garden of Eden. In the center of the dark hole in which I found myself, I held onto this lifeboat of belief which was the foundation of my faith. It stayed with me through weary days and sleepless nights. It helped me make it one moment to the next. It remained in the days of deep desperation and the days of thinking that maybe this time I would get better.

For Karen, the feminine side of faith showed. For some reason, when she came to the bottom of the pit, she knew that Jesus was there in the deep darkness and that he loved her. She hung to this inner belief through the terrible inner storms of the depression and the long nights of insomnia. Somewhere in the center of her being, in the darkest part of her own heart, the Holy Spirit lived. Karen found in the darkness of her own heart of faith, a word, a belief and a lifeboat of Jesus living inside her, of Jesus living in the darkness of her night.

Step IX: The resolution of anger by forgiveness and redirection of the anger

Anger is the disease that spreads itself across the face of the human race like a deadly cancer and perpetuates wars, massacres, murders, and untold human destruction. Unresolved anger regenerates in the form of revenge and retribution. Anger is dangerous in a lethal way to those with depression. People like myself tend to repress and suffocate anger and cause anger to fester and gradually turn itself into the revenge of depression. For other people anger is wielded against another in a forceful and dominating way that produces alienation and isolation for the person with depression.

Forgiveness was for me the first step in healing resentment. Forgiveness helped rid me of perpetual wars that resentment and revenge perpetrate within the psyche. I was still left with the powerful energy of unresolved anger. This was one of the signal causes of the second passage I had through depression. First, I had to learn to become aware of my anger and not deny it no matter how painful it might be. Secondly, I had to learn not to explode in anger either inside or outside myself. To explode on others, something I was personally afraid of, would bring about alienation and isolation. To let anger fester and explode inside myself was so very destructive to me. I had to learn how to become aware of my anger and then learn how to respond and not to react, and how not to turn anger inside myself. Under the guidance of the Holy Spirit I learned to seek the best and most fruitful way to express anger.

How was I to make the truth of what I was feeling the principle issue and not my anger? Over a long period of time I found ways to come to peace and use my emotions of anger to help and energize me to speak the truth. I found that there were hundreds of ways to forcefully express my truth or the offense that I was feeling. Some of the ways that I used to redirect my anger so that it could have a powerful and positive effect included:

1) silence, the refusal to reply,
2) forgiveness,

3) the expression of feeling without judgment,
4) asking the right question
5) understanding the other person first and then responding according to where they were.

The process that I have described for myself was very similar for Karen. In the beginning of her battle with depression, she was unable to admit to herself that she was angry. A long period of therapy enabled her to label her anger and work through it. Later, when she worked with me, we used the process of focusing to enable her to find in her body the signs of anger. She then learned to work through and direct the anger.

Step X: Working through fear by the power of the mystery of Jesus walking on the water

The process of working through fear in a Christian way is found by coming closer to Christ and slowly engaging the grace and virtue of trust in our lives. Learning to trust in God in times of consolation, when we experience the deep presence of God to us, and in the midst of desolation or even the seeming despair of depression is a precious gift; perhaps it is the most precious gift of all. By learning to live by faith in the night or the day of the soul, we can find within us the rock anchored in the Father through Jesus. Trust does not dissolve in the euphoria of consolation or in the desperation of desolation.

This process can best be described as learning how to *walk on water* with Jesus. Like Peter, in order to trust in Jesus and get out of the boat, I ask for the grace to confront my fear, not alone, but with Jesus. As I walk with Peter on the water, I walk in the *now* moment. I am confident that in living in the present, I will receive the grace that is sufficient for survival and recovery.

In each step that I take toward Jesus I ground my faith in him by abandoning myself to him at every moment along the way. Through continuous abandonment of myself to Jesus, an interior connection is formed within my being that remains resiliently present through moments of darkness and moments of light. The resolute abandonment to God in each day and moment of my life slowly forms an interior foundation that does not crack in the face of the most horrendous fear and despair.

For Karen, the movement of the miraculous was most evident in this step. For her, each day was a confrontation with a series of impossibilities she did not think she could face or accomplish. To get up after only a couple of hours sleep, take care of her young daughter, go to work, clean her house, all seemed impossible. By learning how to *walk on the water* and taking Jesus' hand, she was somehow able to perform, what were for her, miraculous actions. Her ability to get up, do her work, take care of her child were daily miracles in her life.

She was able to walk through the fear that she could not do these essential tasks. She was able to hear the admonition of Jesus, "Do not be afraid." Then she was able to break through her fear and terror. With the power of Jesus extending his hand to her across the water she could do the impossible, make her way through strong trials of desolation. In these times she was able to find Jesus even in deep darkness. Her willingness to accept and walk with a life filled with profound physical, psychological, and spiritual desolation enabled her to find Jesus. She found Jesus at the center of the deepest darkness where she walked. To walk on water in the midst of the darkness allowed her to find Jesus in the pitch blackness of the life she was leading.

Step XI: To accept my life one day at a time
In the midst of my own depression I stopped at a window one day, paused, and looked out. I tarried there for a moment or two. That delay allowed the Lord to make a significant change in my struggle. As I peered out the window, I suddenly felt his presence. Jesus was asking me if I could accept this depression. I looked to the many years of desolation that might lie ahead and I firmly replied, "No." "Can you accept this depression one day at a time?" " Yes, I can do that."

In accepting the depression one day at a time, I slowly began to realize that I had been fighting the depression as well as my own life. Though I could not accept the depression itself, (I was not a masochist), I could accept my life one day at a time. Instead of fighting my life I began to enter in and live my life. It is the only life I had and to reject it is to fight my own existence. Not to accept it means to lock myself into depression. I have to live this life. To accept it means to take hold of it, to have hope, and to see into it.

When I regard my life as the enemy, it relates to me as an enemy. Fighting it, it hides itself from me and refuses to reveal anything about itself. So I have little insight into the depression and its causes. When I accept my life and regard it as a friend, I stumble upon the realization that this friend could open up to me and reveal his identity.

The revelation of depression and its inner workings and the ability to see it had some surprising results. I was able to see into my depression and find some of the things that were triggering it. I could clearly see that rejection was a very painful thing for me, something I took deeply to heart. To avoid this pain, I would do anything to get back into the good graces of those who rejected me. I would anticipate who I should be in different relationships. Part of me became a chameleon, turning myself into the most likable color. However, in this process I was, sadly, also rejecting myself. This was the primary cause of my depression on the psychological and spiritual level.

To know the trigger of depression and reveal it to Jesus was a great step forward. Even if the trigger went off, knowing it was a trigger gave me detachment from it. The more I knew it and asked God to heal it, the less powerful it became. Learning to know and accept myself slowly healed some of the origins of the depression.

For Karen the desire to return to a *normal* life had a deep hold upon her. This longing to return to the place one was before the depression began tends to recede as the depression continues. The attempt to return to normality begins to hinder dealing with the abnormal present. Slowly Karen began the practice of accepting, one day at a time, where she was. This acceptance helped her deal with her exhaustion and sleeplessness. It also gave her insight into some of the triggers that were disturbing her life and bringing her mood further down.

One of the things she said to me was that accepting where she was opened her to the truth about herself. In that truth she could face authority figures who often triggered a down time or a depressive moment. Knowing the truth about herself enabled her to stand more firmly in the face of erroneous judgment. This knowledge of herself allowed her to not internalize judgments about her and rejections. (She had to learn that if someone does truly reject you or judge you, that is their sin and not something to feel guilty about or targeted. That rejection or judgment must be left outside oneself and not be taken inside. Without this spear of rejection sticking in a vulnerable place, one can then freely consult Jesus about the truth of the matter.)

Knowing who she was allowed her to stave off the power of those who used oppression against her. It was the truth about herself that set her free. Sometimes she identified a trigger going off in one of her relationships and she could do nothing about it. Just knowing this enabled her to name it and detach from it. Slowly, as her sleeplessness was helped by medication, she saw some triggers defused. Knowing the truth about herself and facing it with Jesus gave her strength to gradually heal part of the depression.

Step XII: Learning how to walk through darkness

Karen had learned how to live with darkness in a powerful way. Though she was a friendly person who prized the intimacy of married life, she was a single mother. She had to constantly live with the fact that the one relationship that might have consoled her in the midst of that loneliness, the relationship of marriage, was denied her. She had learned that the way to deal with loneliness was to face it with Jesus. Walking with the desire for the relationship that she most wanted and sharing with Jesus, she had come to know that Jesus is always with her. Though she had lost the human relationship that she wanted, she penetrated the depth of her own loneliness to find Jesus at the center of that deep darkness.

When one is confronted with the darkness of the spiritual desert, the tendency is to run in fear that God has abandoned you. In the depth of depression the darkness is worse. It has a quality potentially filled with threat or malice. To walk through this foreboding reality seems at first impossible. Somehow Karen had learned to live with this darkness and find her way through the center of it. Contemplative prayer and a constant, unrelenting search for God led her to Jesus in the center of that darkness. The key to the spiritual life in the midst of inner darkness and distress was revealed to her. No matter how deep the darkness, Jesus can be found in the center. In time Karen discovered that through this darkness, Jesus was leading her to the Father.

In her confrontation with the darkness, Karen had learned a truth that St. Paul enunciated so clearly. On earth, we look through a glass darkly (I Cor. 13:12). Despite the consolation that we receive here, there is a darkness that shrouds the face of God. As she walked through the desert and through the terrors of Calvary, Karen was confronted with the dark veil that covers the face of God. Instead of running from it she learned to face it. Like the face suddenly revealed on Veronica's veil, Karen had discovered that Jesus and the Father were found under the dark veil.

Step XIII: Restoration/Reconstruction
Karen still suffered from insomnia and depression. She was taking a moderate dose of antidepressant, that gave her an energy that she had not possessed in the previous years of insomnia and depression. She was then able to take a full-time job. She still experienced relapses, but she had great courage and resourcefulness in making her way through these trying times. She was slowly able to recover her skill as a graphic artist and her abilities blossomed again.

The rebuilding of her life and abilities became evident outwardly and inwardly. We had to wait for God to perform the next miracle in her life, which we were sure God would do because God loved her.

Step XIV: The full growth in the resurrection of Jesus and the desire
to help others in the predicament of depression
Though Karen had experienced something of the resurrection of Jesus in her life, it had not come to full term. Yet, during the time of her struggle, she had been given gifts in the healing ministry. She used these gifts to help people who struggled with depression. As she began to get better, she was able to hone these gifts into a very fine instrument of healing. Her own experience of suffering and desolation was very helpful to others and her compassion for her fellow sufferers was evident.

Final Remarks
Depression is a mysterious disease. In mild depression, one therapeutic

Steps of Recovery from Depression

- Jesus suffered depression before I did.
- The way through depression is one of total surrender for the Christian. In depression I am not alone.
- Live in the present moment. One day at a time. Prepare for the future; do not live in the future.
- If you can take the medication, take it. Be humble and admit you need the help of medication.
- Find the friends who will walk with you without giving advice. Find someone who believes in you and can be a loving mirror.
- Do what you can do; not what you cannot. Find the lifeboats that get you from day to day, from hour to hour, from moment to moment.
- Resurrection thinking - the conclusion of every thought process is realistically positive.
- I was created because God loved me and found me to be good. I was redeemed because God has forgiven me, died for me and restored that original goodness within me.
- Learn how to respond, not how to react. Forgive, pray, and then respond.
- Walk on the water with Jesus. Walk on the now wave. With each step, abandon yourself to Jesus. Slowly confront your fear with Jesus.
- Accept yourself (with depression) one day at a time. As you accept yourself, you can see into yourself. Become aware of your triggers. As time goes on, ask the Lord to heal the triggers.
- My life is one of faith. Whether it be in consolation or desolation, I live in faith. The road through the darkness is the road to my inner self. The road through the darkness is the discovery of the Father.
- The resurrection of Jesus leads to reconstruction. Reconstruction is physical, psychological, and spiritual.
- The resurrection of Jesus leads us to help other depressives.

session, the reading of a self-help book, the facing of the difficulty or trigger, can bring about healing. In Karen's case, the resistance of the body to medication, the severity of side effects, can suffocate the healing process for years.

We have much to learn about depression. It is a disease in which the person must find his/her way on a lonely journey, especially if the symptoms remain resistant to medication or counsel. On this journey the steps we have outlined remain helpful. Each person must find his or her own way out of the pit of depression, battling its manifestations and the negative thinking, to the place where survival becomes recovery.

Attention to one's feelings and emotions and, if one is Christian, attention to the inner voice of conscience are essential to recovery, once into it. It is the suppression of the inner voice, or the ignorance of it that brings about depression in the first place. To block the movement of God is to block the way to health.

On this lonely, often torturous journey, we must deeply respect those with depression, recognizing that we are not their savior, accompanying them along the way, sharing our experience of depression, working the steps together. To show the depressed person our love and our faith in them is most helpful in their attempt to make it from one day to the next.

Reference Notes

Ashbrook, J. B. (1995). *"Psychopharmacology and pastoral counseling: Medication and meaning." The Journal of Pastoral Care, 49 (1):* 5.

Beck, A., Rush, A.J., Shaw, B. and Emery, G. (1979). *The Cognitive Therapy of Depression.* New York: Guilford Press.

Burke, W., (1999). *Protect Us from All Anxiety: Meditations for the Depressed,* Chicago, IL: ACTA Publications.

Burns, D. D., (1980). *Feeling Good*, New York: W. Morrow. The ultimate handbook for cognitive therapy but has it to be watched for non-Christian resolution of ethical problems.

Copeland, M. E., (1992). *The Depression Workbook: A Guide for Living with Depression and Manic Depression,* Oakland, CA: New Harbinger Publications.

Hulme, W. and Hulme, L. (1995). *Wrestling with Depression: A Spiritual Guide to Reclaiming Life.* Minneapolis, MN: Augsburg Fortress Publishers. Some insights from a Christian suffering with depression.

Keating, T. (1994). *Open Mind, Open Heart: The Contemplative Dimension of the Gospel.* Boston, MA: Element Publishing.

McMahon, E. and Campbell, P.A. (1997). *Bio-Spirituality: Focusing as a Way to Grow.* Chicago, IL: Loyola Press.

Mondimore, F. M., (1993). *Depression: The Mood Disease*, Baltimore,

MD: Johns Hopkins University Press.

Pennington, M.B. (1982). *Centering Prayer: Renewing an Ancient Christian Prayer Form.* New York: Image Books.

Styron, W. (1990). *Darkness Visible: A Memoir for Madness.* New York, Random House. Probably the most real description of depression ever written but the author makes his way through depression without God.

Thompson, T., (1995). *The Beast: A Journey Through Depression.* New York: Plume/Penguin. Tracy does not come at this from a Christian perspective but gives a vivid description of depression.

Wheeler, J., (1996). *Gethsemane: From Depression to Hope.* Meditations on depression and the experience of the dark night; the inner healing of finding meaning in depression.

Wheeler, J., (2000). *Why Have You Forsaken Me; Help for Christians Undergoing Depression.* A practical set of steps for a Christian to make his/her way through depression. The latter book is in the process of being published in Spanish. This book and the first book can be obtained by writing to St. Joseph's Prayer Center, 312 Maple Avenue, Patchogue, NY 11772. The suggested donation for *Gethsemane* - fifteen dollars; for *Why* - twenty-five dollars.